Battling Cancer

Hope and Inspiration for the Journey Ahead

PENELOPE CORTEZ

Levers 4 Press

Battling Cancer: Hope and Inspiration for the Journey Ahead
Visit PenelopeCortez.com to access additional resources.
Published by Levers Press, Walnut Creek, California.

Copyright © 2025, Levers Press

The author of this book does not dispense medical advice or prescribe the use of any technique as a form of treatment for physical or medical problems without the advice of a physician, either directly or indirectly. The intent of the author is only to offer information of a general nature to help you in your quest for emotional and spiritual well-being. The information in this book is for general use. In the event you use any of the information in this book for yourself, which is your constitutional right, the author, publisher, and/or copyright owner or licensee assume(s) no responsibility for your actions. The author, publisher, and/or copyright owner or licensee shall not be liable or responsible for any loss, injury or damage allegedly arising from information in this book.

Cover design and interior layout: Victoria Wolf, wolfdesignandmarketing.com
Editors: Megan Ryan and Jennifer Jas

ISBN: 979-8-9917788-0-0
Library of Congress Cataloging-in-Publication Data is available upon request.
Subjects: Health & Fitness / Diseases & Conditions / Cancer / Body, Mind & Spirit / Healing / Prayer & Spiritual / Inspiration & Personal Growth / Religious / Christian Living / Spiritual Growth / Self-Help

Levers 4 Press

Contents

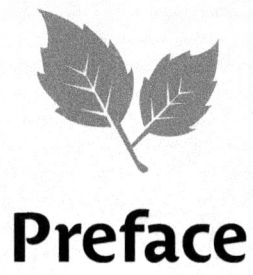

Preface

God gave me a gift. It is called cancer. I remember reading other books that suggested cancer is a gift, and I could not grasp at the beginning of my journey how cancer could be beneficial to anyone.

My cancer journey not only changed my life and how I view the world and the people around me, but it also changed my relationship with God. Proverbs 20:30 (GNT) reinforces this concept when it states, "Sometimes it takes a painful experience to make us change our ways." If you are reading this book, God has already created an opportunity to connect with you through these words. He loves you deeply and wants to help and support you as you fight this disease. This book is a mere vessel to share what God wants you to hear.

Although you do not know how your cancer battle will end, you can decide how you will approach one of the most difficult challenges of your life. I hope that after you read this book, you will have a renewed faith to recognize the miracles that can be found on your cancer journey. I pray that my experiences can bring you hope and inspiration while strengthening your relationship with God.

This book is arranged into five sections: My Journey, Testimonials & Insights, Closing, Reflection & Action, and References.

+ In the first section, entitled My Journey, I will share my cancer story by bringing you into my life and my journey on the road to recovery. I will share challenges and decisions I faced along the way that will help you apply my experiences to your situation.

+ The Testimonials & Insights section summarizes various insights I gained throughout my cancer battle that are key lessons to live by. This section will help you focus your mind, body, and soul on what matters.

- The Closing section summarizes key actions for you to consider as you develop a plan to change your life.

- The Reflection & Action section provides a framework to help you internalize the insights at a deeper level by leaning on Scripture and reflecting on what it means in your life. This section is critical to help you take the concepts provided and turn them into practical action.

- The References section includes recommended reading, a Bible verse bibliography, citations, and sources.

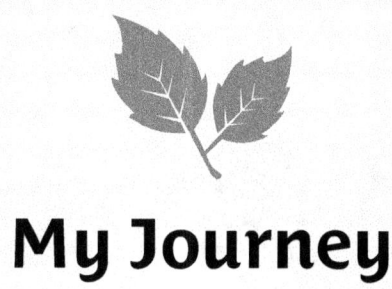

My Journey

Years ago, I remember feeling fortunate because life was going so well. My husband and I faced the typical struggles most families do when raising two children, but overall, life was good.

Work was at the center of my world. I was a self-described workaholic who came from a family of workaholics. I grew up in a home that reinforced strong work ethics, which is admirable; however, this strength turned into a weakness when work became the priority in my life.

I loved solving complex organizational problems and was given the opportunity to advance and hone these skills throughout my career. I considered myself an expert and took pride in what I was able to deliver. I was relentless in my quest to learn, grow, and produce. In one job, I consistently worked ninety hours a week to deliver results. That was the job I held when I was diagnosed with cancer. God sure has a way of reprioritizing our lives and getting our attention.

Despite all my success at work, I never once entertained the concept that I had achieved my accomplishments because God gave me talents, or even because God had given me the chance to develop those talents. I was self-driven and believed that my success was a direct result of how hard I worked. The more I worked, the more I accomplished. The more I accomplished, the more confident I became in my abilities. I never felt that I was arrogant, nor did I boast about my talents to others; however, I did feel that I had an opportunity to embrace humility internally. I recall discussing this desire with my sister. Her wise response was to be careful what you ask for in prayer because God may take you on a journey that you don't expect.

I tried for years to be more humble, with little success. I prayed about it periodically. My perspective and actions didn't substantially change until 2011. Sometimes, we pray for a change, and we don't understand why our prayers are not answered. God was waiting for the right moment when I was ready to grow and handle what it truly means to be humble. There is nothing like facing death to immediately alter how you view your life and who you are as a person. God knew I was finally ready and used cancer to help me change. When I prayed for humility, did I expect to get cancer? Of course not, but God can always bring good out of bad. He used my health challenge to shape my character while answering my prayers.

So how did my cancer journey begin? It was a cold day in November, and I sat by my fireplace to get warm. I folded my arms tightly across my body. Immediately, felt a lump in my right breast. I don't know how, but I absolutely knew the second I felt the lump that it was bad. I was shocked, and I cried immediately. My husband tried to console me by reminding me that we didn't have any information yet on what it could be. But I knew in my heart that something was very wrong.

Different types of cancers permeated my family tree. My aunt and grandmother both had breast cancer. Other cancers in the family were ovarian, skin, and colon. Logically, it was not surprising for me to get cancer, especially given my family history. But the fear that cancer triggers is undeniable. I became intensely focused on getting the appropriate exams scheduled so I could better understand what I was dealing with.

I immediately made an appointment to have an ultrasound. I remember the fear I felt waiting for the doctor to come back with the results. I was by myself when the doctor confirmed I had breast cancer. Even though I had felt sure the test would confirm my worst fear, the shock of hearing I had cancer took me into another dimension.

It was a moment I will never forget. I no longer could hear what people were saying to me or around me. My world forever changed and seemed distant somehow, as if I were looking at it from afar and no longer as an active participant. As the doctor instructed me on the next steps, my mind began to blur. I could not hear what he was saying and just wanted to be at home—a safe, comforting environment with people I loved. I left the office and cried in my car for quite some time before driving back home to tell my family.

Then came all the doctor appointments to properly diagnose the cancer and develop a treatment plan. The amount of information I was expected to process was overwhelming as the various doctors (including an oncologist, radiologist, surgeon, and nutritionist) described their roles in my treatment plan. It was easy to become frustrated since I was still processing the shock of having to deal with cancer. The stress began to mount for obvious reasons, like trying to learn all the new terms and risks, not knowing how cancer would ultimately impact my family and me, and dealing with practical issues, such as having work and family obligations to meet.

I learned that my unique treatment plan required that I make critical decisions that could change the outcome, including whether I would live or die and whether my quality of life would be affected in the short and long term. These decisions became a beacon which helped me navigate through the fog. These decisions gave me back a sense of control and allowed my views, values, and beliefs to shape a plan that worked for me.

Some people assume the doctors will develop the right plan, and they may not know that they have options as patients. Given my problem-solving bias, it was natural for me to look at cancer as a problem that needed to be solved. It was imperative that I research and actively engage in understanding the benefits and risks of each procedure before moving forward. For every benefit that a specific treatment provided, there was always a downside, so being informed was critical. Some of my decisions were:

- Should I participate in genetic testing?
- Should I choose a lumpectomy or mastectomy?
- Should I pursue chemotherapy? If so, do I want a port installed?
- Should I go through radiation?
- Should I take medication to reduce the risk of reoccurrence, and if so, for how long?

As I faced the various decisions, I moved emotionally from denial to shock and then to acceptance. The decisions that needed to be made meant I could no longer avoid the fact that I had cancer, and I needed information to ensure I was making the best choices. I spent months gathering information to better understand my cancer and the benefits and risks associated with the various treatment options. Later, I realized that all those talents I used at work were the same talents I used to ensure I had the right treatment plan. It became clear to me that God had a far bigger purpose for the gifts he had helped me develop at work. The importance of thanking God for my unique talents became even clearer as I could rely on those skills to gather the right information despite being emotionally and physically exhausted.

My cancer was described as invasive ductal carcinoma and estrogen receptor (ER) positive, which meant my naturally occurring estrogen was stimulating my cancer growth. The cancer was classified as Stage 2 (the tumor was more than two centimeters but less than five centimeters). In reviewing the ultrasound report, I saw that the radiologist described the tumor as slow-growing. I could not grasp this conclusion nor accept it. I wondered how a cancerous lump could be slow-growing if it had not shown up on the annual mammogram screening the previous year. I was reassured by the doctors that the cancer was slow growing. Despite this, I felt the need to act quickly to remove the underlying tumor as soon as possible, given how fast I thought it was growing and that it might be spreading to other body parts. I was so thankful to have an expert oncologist with me every step of the way who helped guide me through the various decisions while providing emotional support. I believe God brought us together so I could benefit from her deep compassion for and skills in treating breast cancer patients.

Because my cancer tumor was relatively small, I considered having a lumpectomy rather than a mastectomy. Given my family history of breast and ovarian cancer, it was not a decision I took lightly. I was given the opportunity to do genetic testing. This testing would allow me to understand if I had the BRCA (BReast CAncer) gene. If the gene is present, an individual is predisposed to breast cancer. In fact, according to the National Cancer Institute at the time this book was written, "55%–72% of women who inherit a harmful *BRCA1* variant and 45%–69% of women who inherit a harmful *BRCA2* variant will develop breast cancer by 70–80 years of age."[1]

Given the high cancer rate of those with a BRCA variant, I decided it was essential for me to know if I had this gene before I made my final decision on the type of surgery I would pursue—a lumpectomy or a mastectomy. A lumpectomy removes only the impacted tissue, so it is less aggressive than a mastectomy, which removes the entire breast and is a much more complex surgery and recovery. Thankfully, genetic testing showed I did not have this gene, which confirmed my decision that a lumpectomy was the best course of action.

Thirty minutes prior to going into surgery to have a lumpectomy, I was given a test where a dye was injected into my lymphatic system. This dye shows if the cancer cells have spread to the lymph nodes. If cancer reaches the lymphatic system, it can spread more easily throughout the body. I learned through this test that the cancer had already spread to my lymph nodes. I had nine lymph nodes removed during surgery as a result of this new finding.

So I bring you back to the statement from the radiologist that the cancer was slow-growing. The fact that the cancer had already reached my lymph nodes confirmed, at least in my mind, that this cancer was actually growing quickly. If I had waited, the cancer may have spread throughout my lymphatic system, and the outcome could have been very different for me.

I knew then that my assessment of the situation was correct, and I am thankful I acted quickly rather than waiting. Finding out that the cancer had reached my lymph nodes suggested a more aggressive approach to the next steps of my treatment plan.

While it is critical to listen to and rely on medical expertise, it is also critical that you conduct your own research and listen to what your body and God are telling you. God created the human body, which has its own mechanisms to provide data that should not be ignored. Being attuned to your body, listening to experts, and asking for God's guidance are key steps to ensure you are making the right decisions.

My surgery went well. My surgeon was excellent and left just a two-inch scar. However, that little scar masked the full breadth of healing that needed to occur. With any surgery, scar tissue develops. What I did not realize is how much scar tissue hurts. Once the skin healed, I was diligent in performing daily self-massage to break down the scar tissue and increase the blood flow to the area. I also used oils on the incision scar to reduce the redness and prevent the development of keloids or the excessive growth of fibrous tissue that could increase the size and depth of the scar.

There were two side effects of having some lymph nodes removed. One side effect is called lymphedema, which my doctor discussed with me as a potential risk. Lymphedema is swelling due to the build-up of lymph fluid in the body.[2] The removal of lymph nodes disrupts the flow of lymph, which can lead to swelling. It brought back memories of my aunt who died of breast cancer. She had a huge, swollen arm before she passed. I was diligent in doing a postoperative massage and kept a watchful eye on any swelling. I also wore a compression sleeve when traveling by airplane, as changes in cabin pressure could trigger the swelling. To this day, I feel fortunate that I never experienced lymphedema as a result of my lymph nodes being removed.

The second side effect was never highlighted as a risk by my doctors but did occur a few months after surgery. When I lifted my arm, I noticed a cord or band under my skin that ran from my armpit to my elbow. When

I extended my arm, it felt like this band would snap, and it was uncomfortable. I wasn't sure at the time if it was a tendon or a ligament. Through research, I learned the condition is called *cording*.[3] I discovered an online video that highlighted exercises and massage techniques to gain arm and shoulder movement. Although I am unable to find the specific video I used since it was so many years ago, I encourage you to do a quick search online on this topic and talk with your doctor if you are facing this condition.

After diligently doing the exercises described in the video, the cord disappeared, and I regained mobility in my arm. The individual in the video showed kindness and care by taking the time to share a lesson to help others, which reinforces for me just how much we need each other to get through life's challenges. This is also another example of why it is important to use all your resources during your recovery, including checking in with your physician to ensure the steps you take are appropriate and beneficial.

After the surgery, I decided to leverage chemotherapy (commonly referred to as chemo), radiation therapy, and medication (to suppress estrogen, which was the fuel that the cancer cells used to grow) as part of my postoperative treatment plan. Although the doctor felt confident the cancer had not spread beyond my lymph nodes, I did not feel as assured. I was determined to stop any cancer that may have spread elsewhere in my body, so as a precautionary measure, I selected a more aggressive approach to treatment. I was confident in this decision and my ability to deal with the downsides of radiation, chemo, and medication to ensure no cancer remained. If I was going to battle cancer, I wanted to battle it only once.

After I healed from surgery and completed my exercises and massage, I began chemotherapy and then radiation therapy. While some people dread these therapies, I embraced them because I believed they were essential to my long-term health, especially if the cancer had escaped and was spreading through my lymph system. While these therapies were mitigating my risk of cancer reoccurrence, I began to reframe the problem I was solving. I was no longer sick, as the surgery had rid my body of the cancer. I constantly reminded myself that the cancer was gone, and I must now turn my focus to my health. My treatment plan became my health plan.

Chemotherapy and radiation are choices, and I believed they were essential components to ensure I remained healthy. From that point on, I never associated treatments with being a cancer patient in recovery; rather, I needed these treatments to ensure my health and well-being.

When I started chemotherapy, I was informed that any injections needed to be on the opposite side of where my cancer had been removed. Unfortunately, the arm I was supposed to use to receive the chemo cocktail (a mix of chemo-related chemicals) had very small veins. Every appointment started with excruciating pain as nurses often tried multiple times to insert the needle in the vein properly. It was hard to maintain a positive, upbeat approach to treatment when the anxiety and dread of facing this pain mounted every time I received the chemo treatment.

Given the pain this activity caused, I was offered the option to install a port, which is surgically implanted into your chest and would make it very easy to administer the chemo—no more needles. Although the benefits of skipping ongoing pain at each treatment were appealing, I learned from a colleague who had faced cancer that the port location could get infected, cause other issues, and leave a large scar. I decided that having pain a couple of times a week was better than having a lifelong scar and other potential complications.

The nurses eventually switched to using a needle that's typically used for babies, and the treatments became more bearable. This is another example of seeking out information from others who have gone through a similar trial to help you better understand the benefits and risks so you can make the best choice.

Once I started the chemo phase, as mentioned earlier, my focus turned to health and well-being. As the chemo cocktail dripped down the various tubes and into my veins, I would read inspirational messages, thanking God for helping me through the process. I selected a specific chair placed by a window for each treatment. I would focus my attention on the beautiful trees, which created a calming and tranquil environment as I received the drugs. I brought mementos given to me by family and friends, and they reminded me of the support I had. I felt so fortunate to have my husband sit with me through every session. I reinforced in my mind that each chemo treatment was a positive experience, given it was a tool in my health plan.

When I got home from each appointment, my goal was to rid my body of the toxins. My belief (which is not based on any specific data that I gathered) was that chemo would kill any remaining cancer cells upon contact but could also damage my healthy organs and tissues. It was critical to me to rid my body of the chemo toxins as quickly as possible. I felt this strategy would allow me to get all the benefits of chemo and mitigate the treatment risks to my healthy body parts.

While my body was working overtime trying to heal and rest, I relied on my mind, guided by God's will, to encourage me to move and hydrate even when I did not want to. While I felt like sitting down and resting, I forced myself to walk as soon as I got home, and I drank tons of water immediately following each chemo treatment. After a few days of walking, I would have more energy, so I would exercise more extensively, trying to build up a sweat while doing so. When I worked out, I would talk to my body directly about how proud I was that it was fighting to get me healthy, and I committed to doing my part to ensure I stayed focused and positive while my body was doing the work of healing. God, your inner voice, and positive visualization can be powerful weapons in helping you face the various obstacles in your life.

Although I did not always feel well after the treatments, I reminded myself during those times that I was no longer sick from cancer. If I was not sick, I would not look sick. I visualized the benefits of chemo, including how the chemo attacked the cancer and resulted in a rebirth as my healthy cells were rejuvenated. I encouraged my body to heal and thanked it for doing what was necessary to achieve health. I exercised and focused on nutrition, visualization, and prayer. I had been given another chance at life, and I was absolutely thankful for this gift.

I distinctly remember when my hair started to fall out after several chemo treatments. I found myself holding a handful of hair in the shower. The texture of my hair also started to change. At one point, I looked in the mirror and felt like one of those mangy, unkempt mutts you may see running around the streets of a developing nation. At that point, I asked one of my daughters to help me shave my head because I thought my hair made me look unhealthy and gave the perception that I was sick, which was not what I believed or wanted to convey to others.

For women, especially, losing their hair can be traumatic. For me, it was just part of the process that I was prepared for. The American Cancer Society offers many services to individuals who are battling cancer. I took advantage of their wig services. My sister came with me as I tried on different options, and she helped me select two wigs, as well as some hats and scarves. When I arrived home, I showed my husband the two wigs I had selected. His response crushed me, as he didn't like either of them.

Wearing a wig did not feel natural to me. I wore them just a few times and felt so self-conscious for two reasons. First, I felt people were staring at me, knowing it was a wig. I kept trying to tell myself that many people wear and change wigs as a fashion statement, but I never felt comfortable in them. Second, I felt I was telling the world I was ashamed in some way, that I was hiding because I did not want people to know I had cancer. By wearing a wig or head scarf, I felt I was hiding what I was going through, which didn't feel real or authentic—it felt like a façade. I could never shake those feelings.

Before you pass judgment on my husband and conclude that he wasn't supportive of my wig choices, I must share the context. My husband has shown me every day of our marriage how much he loves me. He loves me for who I am. He has never cared about how I have aged or what I look like. In his way, when he expressed his opinion about the wigs, he meant I was beautiful just as I was. He saw no reason for me to use a wig or scarf. He loved me for me even if I was bald.

After just a few outings wearing either wigs or scarves, I decided I would hang up my wigs and be bald and proud. From that moment, I let go of the notion of having to wear a wig or scarf, which brought a renewed confidence. Everyone is different; however, I felt stronger and healthier by showing the world who I was and that cancer was not going to stop me from living or result in me hiding behind an object that masked the severity of the disease. When I went out clearly showing the full shape of my bald head, I made it a point to dress nicely and accessorize. I never saw myself as a frail, sick person going through chemo with a bald head but rather as a person who had confidence and was enjoying life and just happened to be bald.

The way I presented myself impacted the people around me. Strangers would stop me in the stores and offer me words of wisdom or comfort. One neighbor I hadn't seen in years drove by my house as I was gardening, stopped her car, jumped out, and hugged me. It never occurred to me that my personal choice to go bald would have such a positive and profound effect on others. I realized how this one act created opportunities for me and others to show grace, humility, and compassion. I recognized that I might be triggering an emotional response in someone I did not know just by walking near them. While initially, going bald had helped me and my confidence, I came to realize how my actions impacted others in positive ways that I had not anticipated. This was yet another gift that brought me joy and happiness.

My radiation treatments started right after I completed chemo. I had radiation therapy every day for six weeks. Because of the exposure and impact on my skin, I was diligent to follow the doctor's guidance to lotion the radiated areas two or three times a day after treatment.

Radiation technologists are trained to set up the machines to ensure the radiation treatment is targeted. Yet, after a few sessions, the lung below the treatment area began to hurt and I had trouble breathing. I expressed my concern to the technologist. Although he reinforced that the radiation was not reaching my lung, he did recheck the settings. He assured me that the radiation treatment should not cause breathing issues. However, I continued to have trouble breathing during and sometimes after the treatments. The doctors could not explain why and, in some ways, discounted my concerns.

While going through radiation treatments and struggling with breathing, I started having strange dreams about breathing. Almost nightly, I would dream that if air went down the wrong tube, I would die. I would wake up in sheer panic, thinking I was going to die because I breathed the wrong way while sleeping. It was terrifying because it felt so real. We all know dreams can be irrational. Despite knowing this and telling myself daily that what I was dreaming was not reality, I continued to have these dreams and associated panic attacks for almost a year. This was another mental and physical side effect that I did not understand or anticipate.

Another unexpected outcome of radiation was that my chest bones that were exposed to radiation hurt when touched. I was told by my oncologist that the pain would likely never fully go away. More than a decade later, I can attest that she was right. I still have minor pain when my bones are touched, primarily in the sternum and upper ribs.

When I completed chemo and radiation, I moved to the next phase, which was to suppress my estrogen through daily medication. Like any drug, there are side effects. I felt fortunate I was able to tolerate tamoxifen, as I discovered through research that many people have significant and painful side effects from this drug. When I was first prescribed the medication, my oncologist showed me data that highlighted how tamoxifen was successful in preventing a reoccurrence of my type of cancer if taken for five years. When the five-year milestone came, new research suggested a significant reduction in reoccurrence of cancer if the drug is taken for ten years. Based on this data, I agreed to take the medication for ten years.

Looking back, I realize I ultimately traded the benefits of maintaining estrogen levels for reducing the risk of cancer reoccurrence. Because I didn't have side effects while taking the drug, I did not fully appreciate the potential long-term effect it would have on my skin and bones. Today, I believe I aged prematurely as a result of suppressing my estrogen for so many years. I also have some bone loss, which is a side effect of this drug. In retrospect, I should have taken the medication for the first five years to reduce reoccurrence but then allowed my body to stabilize while I could still produce estrogen.

There are always trade-offs that need to be considered as you develop a treatment plan that works for you. You will have to make decisions based on the best information you have at the time, as you will never have perfect information. I acknowledge this is one choice I would have changed. When I look in the mirror, I can't help but be reminded of my cancer journey. I continue to remind myself that there is no value in second-guessing decisions already made; the value is in learning from them. From a lessons standpoint, I believe some of the steps I took in the areas of mindset, nutrition, and exercise helped me mitigate some of the drug's side effects. From a medication perspective, I should have considered the potential long-term impact more carefully.

Cancer and its associated treatments—such as chemo, radiation, and medication—are hard on your body. Given this, most treatment plans include guidance on what to eat and drink and what types of exercise are appropriate. However, adopting these suggestions can be hard. It often requires changing your mindset about the role of food and exercise in your life. The way you think and what you value will shape how well you leverage these three fundamental levers to help you heal.

I will share some of my beliefs that kept me focused and helped me realize the true benefits of changing one's mindset and approaching food, drink, and exercise differently. As you consider your own adjustments, please consult with your doctors and specialists to ensure you understand the benefits and risks of any changes you want to make, given your specific health challenges.

Mindset

Your thoughts can impact your health. A mindset is a set of beliefs or attitudes that shape your view of the world and yourself. Your attitudes can influence your emotions. You have a choice in how you respond to positive and negative emotions. Negative emotions—such as anger, fear, frustration, and cynicism—can be expected periodically during your journey, but a continued focus on negativity can impact your recovery. In contrast, positive emotions, such as gratitude and thankfulness, can help you in your recovery and bring lifelong peace and joy.

When hearing the word *cancer*, you will undoubtedly be shocked, and it will take time for you to process your situation and what you are dealing with. However, it is vital that you don't fall into a victim mentality. I never questioned why I got cancer or asked, "Why me?" In fact, I felt, "Why not me?" The American Cancer Society states there is a one in eight chance a woman will develop breast cancer.[4] Given my family history of breast cancer, there was a high probability that I, my mom, or one of my sisters would get breast cancer. Don't waste precious time by focusing on the past nor why you have cancer. Focus on making the changes you need to make today to alter the rest of your life.

One mindset to think about is how you perceive your illness and God's role in it. God is always good and will not hurt you. You may get sick from factors you can control, such as not living a healthy lifestyle, or circumstances you cannot control, such as environmental hazards or damaged genes or DNA. However, God can always turn a bad situation into something good if you trust him. A wise pastor once said that God can use illness in various ways including:[5]

1. To teach us or to help us grow. Psalm 119:71 (NLT) says, "My suffering was good for me, / for it taught me to pay attention to your decrees." In my case, I prayed for humility for years but did not change until I faced my battle with cancer. I was also focused on the wrong priorities for most of my adult life. Cancer helped me reprioritize what I value and how I spend my time and resources.

2. To bring glory to God. Glory to God can happen when you are healed and testify to others about God's healing power, or when you are not healed, yet you stay true to God through your pain and suffering. I wrote this book to bring glory to God through words that can bring hope and inspiration to others.

God used my cancer in so many ways. Cancer helped me learn to be more humble, to have more compassion for others, to embrace the goodness and blessings in life daily, to fully trust God and his plan for my life, and to bring glory to him through sharing my experiences.

What you believe to be true will shape how you think, the actions you take, how you spend your time, and how you treat others. Positive messages can shift your mindset by helping you reflect on and be thankful for today while giving you a pathway to change for tomorrow.

Before I wrap up the topic of mindset, I would like to delve deeper into my mindset about genetic testing. Genetic testing has continued to evolve since I was given the opportunity to participate in 2012. Although the BRCA gene is one of the earliest genes identified related to breast cancer, other gene mutations that can influence one's breast cancer risk have been discovered since I was tested.[6] You may have another type of cancer, so it is imperative to understand whether there are gene mutations associated with your cancer that could impact your treatment plan. Understanding your cancer risk and the availability of genetic information is an important step in developing your treatment options.

Given the advancements in genetic testing, I have been encouraged by my oncologist in the last few years to participate in more extensive genetic tests beyond breast cancer. I have declined these tests because of my mindset and what I believe to be true about how they would impact me. My oncologist discussed the benefits of detailed genetic testing, including knowing what diseases I may be predisposed to so I can make adjustments to my lifestyle. My doctor also talked about the value of this information for my children so they, too, can make changes.

While I don't debate these benefits, I believe there is significantly more downside than upside if I obtain this additional genetic information. My rationale is:

1. This data wouldn't influence any decision I need to make currently.

2. I maintain a fairly healthy lifestyle, so I am not sure what else I or my children would do with this information.

3. I actually don't want to know all the diseases I may get. In fact, just because you have a specific gene that predisposes you to a disease does not guarantee that you will get that disease. Having

this information would fill my mind with worry, which, in turn, can cause disease. It can become a self-fulfilling prophecy. You think you will get sick, so you will get sick. I don't want to live life worrying about what might happen.

I believe genetic screening is extremely helpful if it will change your treatment plan and if the benefit of having the information outweighs the risk of not having it. If you live an unhealthy lifestyle, you can easily do research to understand what diseases you may get, and you can make changes without the genetic information; however, if you are someone who needs that extra push to change, maybe you should pursue this type of testing. You know yourself more than anyone else, so consider the benefits and risks of genetic testing, given your mindset, beliefs, and likelihood of taking action on the information before you proceed.

Diet and Exercise

What you eat can either help or hinder your progress. I followed the guidance of my nutritionist by eating healthy and incorporating significant protein into my diet. Protein is crucial as cells are recovering, rejuvenating, and replicating after chemo and radiation. One critical role you must play is to give your body what it needs so it can recover. This is one of the levers you have complete control over. Our bodies want to heal. God not only gave us these capabilities, but he also gave us specific foods that can enable healing. The choices you make about what to put into your body before, during, and after your treatments matter. Choosing highly nutritionally dense foods will empower your healing.

If you don't have a nutritionist—or even if you do—consider reading the myriad of published books that will guide you on how to eat during and after your treatments. In the References section, I have listed a few books that I read during my journey. I can't thank the authors of these books enough for taking the time to share their thoughts which helped me heal. My book is a testament to them as I try to help you in the same way they helped me.

I am in no way an expert on nutrition or exercise, but I believe that what I ate and drank and how I incorporated exercise had a tremendous effect on how I felt during treatment and how I recovered after treatment. During my chemo treatments, nausea was minimal. During the chemo phase, I actually felt better than I had felt most of my life, and I attribute that to my diet and exercise plan.

During your treatment cycles, consider my personal tips, which I picked up through the books I listed and other general research:

Tip #1 Water: Drink plenty of water before and during your treatment: at least sixteen ounces before and eight ounces during. After your treatment, drink eight ounces or more of liquids every hour to flush out the toxins. I drank seventy to eighty ounces a day. Add fresh lemon to your water, as lemon strengthens the immune system and cleanses the stomach. In addition, if you are experiencing a metal taste in your mouth after chemo treatment, drinking more water will help the metal taste subside faster.

Drinking all this water means you will spend a lot of time in the bathroom urinating. Urinating is one way to dispose of some of the chemicals. Keep in mind that because the chemo chemicals may be present in your urine, you should take extra care to flush the toilet with the cover down, as some toilets actually spray some of the toilet bowl contents into the air, and you don't want to inhale any chemicals you just disposed of.

Tip #2 Exercise: The other way to rid yourself of the chemo chemicals is to sweat them out through exercise. I made a commitment to exercise after each treatment, even when I did not feel like it. If you have put in the effort to achieve an exercise goal, you probably have experienced a time when you didn't feel like working out. However, when you push through it, you realize you can do more than anticipated. Leverage your mind, your determination, and the power of prayer to give you the push to exercise when you don't want to.

With chemo, your body will be tired and you may be sick, so your body will tell you to sit down and rest. For me, rest meant I was not doing my part to help my body heal. I believed every minute of delay meant I was allowing chemicals to potentially hurt other organs or tissues, which would harm me in the long term. I had full control of my decision to exercise or not, so it was up to me to help my body. It became an absolute necessity to work out if I didn't want chemo to damage other parts of my body. Not exercising was not an option.

With that said, you may not have a lot of strength or stamina, so aggressive exercise may not be an option immediately following treatment. Do try and push yourself, and you will discover you can do more than you thought. For me, after each treatment, I typically walked one to three miles and tried to walk at a pace that triggered a sweat. Getting outdoors also gave me a chance to embrace nature and God's healing presence during my walks.

Tip #3 Eating: On the day of my chemo treatment, I often didn't eat much—not because of feeling nauseous, which I sometimes did, but because I just didn't feel like eating. What I ate became vital to me, as my choices could help my body heal. God gave us many foods and spices to help us repair our own bodies, and I tried to leverage nutritionally dense foods that had healing qualities. As I read the books mentioned in the Recommended Reading section and embraced healthy eating, I was amazed at how wonderful I felt: I was less hungry, and I lost weight easily.

Here are a few actions to consider as part of your healthy eating plan:

1. *Eat organic foods when possible.* With this said, even organic foods may contain natural pesticides and a few synthetic pesticides approved for organic farming. It is essential to check labels. Organic foods are preferred, as they contain fewer additives and preservatives compared to nonorganic foods, but you may never eliminate all these additives from your diet. The premise is to minimize pesticides and animal hormones in your body whenever possible while your cells are rejuvenating. It's true that organic foods are more expensive, so you may need to prioritize which organic foods you select, given your food budget. A good rule of thumb is this: If a fruit or vegetable has a thick skin that will be removed, such as bananas or avocados, you can buy nonorganic, as you will peel and discard the skin that was exposed to the chemicals. If you are eating the entire fruit or vegetable, choose organic.

2. *Consume significant amounts of protein.* Protein is critical when recovering. To minimize exposure to animal hormones and antibiotics, select organic meats. Beef and chicken are often injected with hormones or antibiotics. Although I'm not a vegetarian, I do

not eat much beef or chicken. Trying to figure out how to consume forty-five to sixty grams of protein per day was a challenge. Ask your doctor to help guide you on the appropriate amount and types of protein to consume while going through treatment. To boost my daily protein intake, I mixed protein powder into my smoothies, drank high-protein milk, added nutritional yeast to my meals, and ate lots of eggs, beans, and lentils.

3. *Eat fresh food whenever possible* (no processed foods or foods with preservatives). Focus on foods that give you the most nutrition. Fresh foods will also help you lower your sugar and fat consumption. Frozen fruits and vegetables have less nutrition than their fresh counterparts, as they lose some of their vitamins and minerals during production.

4. *Avoid canned food if possible.* Research from the National Institute of Environmental Health Sciences states that the chemical bisphenol A (BPA) can leach into food from the epoxy resin coatings of canned foods.[7] Although the Can Manufacturers Institute (CMI) says most canned food no longer contains BPA,[8] can liners still contain other chemicals you want to avoid. You do not need chemicals in your body while you are healing. Do your own research on this topic to decide what is best for you.

5. *Reduce or eliminate refined or processed sugar.* I limited my daily sugar intake to forty to fifty grams per day, which included natural foods that contained some sugar. Sugar is in many foods, including fruit. Reading labels became part of my daily routine. Because I made smoothies daily that contained fresh apple juice and berries in addition to the protein powder that had a few grams of sugar, I

never could eliminate sugar entirely, as the health benefits of the fruits and protein powder outweighed the risk of consuming a small amount of sugar.

I avoided manufactured sugars because they are artificial and may have an impact on health, including increasing the risk of Type 2 diabetes, cardiovascular diseases, and weight gain.[9,10] Do research on the side effects and potential impacts of artificial sugars such as sucralose (Splenda), saccharin (Sweet'N Low), aspartame (NutraSweet, Equal), and stevia (Truvia, Pure Via). To this day, I choose not to consume artificial sugar because of the health risks.

6. *Avoid alcohol.* I gave up alcohol for almost two years. The toughest part of giving up alcohol was the socializing aspect. I initially felt uncomfortable going out to a bar or restaurant since alcohol is so intertwined with how we engage with others. I discovered that carbonated water or seltzer with a splash of cranberry was a perfect drink for these occasions. I developed a new respect and appreciation for nondrinkers and the difficulties they face in a society that is centered around alcohol.

I have provided a sampling of meals below that incorporate the prior suggestions, as well as additional herbs and supplements to boost nutrition and healing.

Breakfast

+ **Hot Cereal:** Enjoy a warm and soothing breakfast, such as oatmeal or Bob's Red Mill Organic Creamy Wheat Hot Cereal.

- **Eggs and Nuts:** Consume protein in the morning with one to two scrambled eggs or one hard-boiled egg along with pepitas or pumpkin seeds, a few walnuts, and a few almonds. This remains my go-to breakfast.

- **Fruit Smoothie:** Consider a smoothie for breakfast or a midmorning snack. You can find smoothie recipes online. Here is one recipe I used frequently: Juice two apples. Place fresh apple juice in blender, add your berries of choice and a cup of ice. Add one scoop of protein power and one cup of super greens. Add a few liquid drops of milk thistle and echinacea to boost your immune system and detox your liver.

Your liver may be under extensive stress as a result of chemo or other medications you may be taking.[11] A 2020 study highlighted in the National Library of Medicine concluded that milk thistle may help protect the liver from chemo damage.[12] Echinacea helps boost your immune system. You can get milk thistle and echinacea at any herbal or natural food store. I've read that aloe vera can help, too, so you can add it to your juice, although I didn't like the taste of it. Always read the benefits and risks and talk to your doctor before taking any supplements.

Lunch

- **Salads/Soups:** TruRoots offers highly nutritious organic products that can be used in salads or soups.

- **Drinks:** Drink at least sixty to seventy ounces of water daily. I supplemented with eleven ounces of high-protein milk, such as Muscle Milk, during lunch, with the sole purpose of boosting my protein intake. Although high-protein milk may contain artificial ingredients, I chose to drink it, as it provided twenty grams of protein with only one hundred calories. Eating protein is essential as your cells are rejuvenating. However, eating a lot of protein can make you gain weight, especially if you're a woman. High-protein milk helped me maintain weight while giving me much-needed protein.

Dinner

+ **Legumes/Beans:** Highly nutritious dried whole beans, including pinto, black, red, garbanzo, and lentils, can be served warm or cold. Consider making soups with a bean base and incorporating onions, nutritional yeast, and dried seaweed (arame, nori, wakame, and kombu), which contains many antioxidants and nutrients.

+ **Other Proteins:** Periodically bake or sauté chicken or a hamburger patty for a good protein boost.

+ **Rice/Grains:** On treatment day, try rice or quinoa. Sauté onions and add Trader Joe's Salsa Autentica, which contains no preservatives. Then add the quinoa or bulgur, a highly nutritious wheat, and boil for about twenty minutes. I refrain from frequently eating rice, as both organic and nonorganic rice contain some level of arsenic, which is cancer-causing.

+ **Vegetables:** Fresh raw or warm vegetables, either baked or sautéed, are an excellent way to consume important nutrients. Incorporating ingredients such as mushrooms, onions, ginger, garlic, and turmeric into recipes is an easy way to boost your immune system.

Snacks/Desserts

+ **Fresh fruits** such as berries and apples are a good snack choice. Sprinkle with cinnamon, which is a natural anti-inflammatory.

+ **Vegetables** such as carrots and cauliflower are highly nutritious. Splurge by allowing yourself to dip the vegetables in organic ranch dressing.

+ **Nuts** such as almonds or walnuts have many health benefits and can curb hunger. Avoid nuts high in saturated fats, such as cashews, Brazil nuts, and macadamia nuts. Avoid peanuts because they are higher in saturated fats and phosphorus, which can limit your body's absorption of other minerals like zinc and iron.

+ **Organic chocolate pudding** is a great treat if you are feeling the need for a sweet dessert.

+ **Dates** are high in fiber and antioxidants. Enjoy this highly nutritious fruit by removing the date nut, rolling in a ball, and coating with cocoa powder and nuts.

Additional foods and spices to consider for their health benefits:

+ **Organic garlic and onions** can cut the risk of stomach cancer in half, according to a Chinese research study.[13]

+ **Organic arame** is a seaweed that helps detox the body. You can add it to soups or to your bean trio salad (after you cook it).

+ **Organic mushrooms** help boost your immune system and have anti-tumor effects. Mushrooms have AHCC (active hexose correlated compound), which protects the immune system from the depressing effects of chemo and reduces side effects.

+ **Organic grapes** have resveratrol and phytochemicals that are found to have anti-inflammatory, antiplatelet, and anticarcinogenic effects.

+ **Organic cruciferous vegetables** such as broccoli and cauliflower are high in isothiocyanates, which activate enzymes present in cells that detoxify carcinogens.

+ **Organic turmeric** helps with inflammation, kidney health, and anxiety.

+ **Organic kukicha tea** helps alkalize the body. To function properly, your body should have a balanced pH (potential hydrogen). Sickness, disease, and cancer often grow when your body is unbalanced. You can purchase pH strips online to test your urine and pH levels.

+ **Organic ginger** is another anti-inflammatory food. Mix it in your soups, salads, or other recipes. Ginger also can help mitigate nausea, reduce pain, and improve digestion and brain function.

One of the books I read recommended taking a ginger bath after treatment due to its healing properties. I discovered a good soak in a tub with ginger has soothing benefits for the body and mind. I also felt that the ginger bath helped with the detoxification process after each treatment. I took a ginger bath every other day plus every day when I had treatment.

To prepare the ginger for a bath, peel ginger and dice it into small pieces. Place diced ginger into a tea mesh ball. Fill a small pot with water, place the mesh ball with ginger in the water, and boil. Just like a traditional tea, the water becomes infused with ginger. Remove the mesh ball, and discard the ginger. Take the pot of infused ginger water and pour it into a bathtub of warm water. Relax and enjoy.

I encourage you to do your own research to discover what foods and spices can improve your health.

Exercise

We all intuitively know that exercise is good for us. Research has shown that exercise boosts your immunity. Cancer.org mentions exercise as especially valuable for cancer patients, as it can reduce fatigue, anxiety, and depression, and it can increase self-esteem and happiness.[14] Working out can help you get rid of the chemo chemicals in your body through sweat and can help with your overall well-being.

During treatment, always remember that your body needs you. Your body will do everything in its power to heal naturally, but you can help it. You must take control and help your body recover. You are stronger than cancer, so force yourself to get off the couch. Ask God in prayer to give you support and the strength to exercise when you do not want to.

Set a goal to sweat every day. Find a physical activity that you enjoy. I walked two miles after breakfast and then again after lunch. I also lifted weights to help my muscles. Your exercise routine may vary and should be guided by your treatment plan.

Part of your plan should include getting outside and enjoying nature. Nature has a way of healing the mind, body, and soul. A 2019 study conducted by the European Centre for Environment & Human Health at the University of Exeter confirmed that spending 120 minutes a week outside with nature was associated with good health and well-being.[15] When you look at the sky, stars, trees, mountains, fields, grass, and clouds with wonderment and awe, you, too, will feel the power of God's sovereignty and the healing power of nature.

In this section, I have shared various tips for implementing food, hydration, and exercise changes, as well as visualization and positive affirmation and support techniques through self-talk and prayer. After implementing all these changes, I can attest that I felt the healthiest I have ever felt in my lifetime. I encourage you to use your cancer journey to learn to lean on God, your mind and body, and resources (such as nature, food, doctors, and research) to help you during the most difficult time in your life.

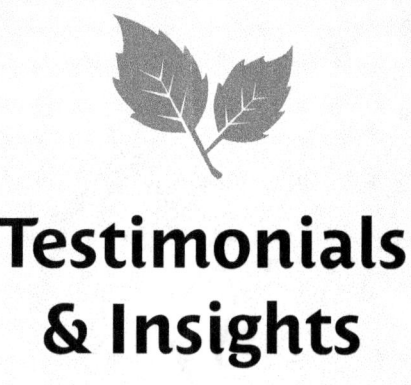

Testimonials
& Insights

Lessons to Live By

With all the challenges that come with battling cancer, you can easily miss the work God is doing in your life; as you are busy confronting the physical and mental impacts of the disease. In this section, you will gain a deeper appreciation for specific events, situations, and experiences in which God works in our lives in ways that can benefit others. I call these my testimonials, as they are at the heart of how God worked in my life to change my perspective and how I see myself and others. Each testimony includes an insight or key takeaway from my experience that I hope you can apply to your situation.

The following table summarizes the insights or takeaways from ten different testimonials I experienced during my yearlong battle with cancer.

#	Insights
1	Mindset: Cancer doesn't define you
2	Character: Managing emotion grows character
3	Faith: I am not alone
4	Empathy: Caring for others brings joy
5	Petition: Prayer is powerful and comforting
6	Guidance: God speaks to us in many ways
7	Support: Resources are provided at the right time
8	Forgiveness: Grace gives us the power to forgive
9	Gratitude: Humility changes how we view life
10	Love: Seeing goodness in others is transformative

I have described the situations, mindsets, and behaviors in each testimonial that, with God's help, became the catalysts for reshaping my perspective in these ten key areas. As you reflect on your situation, mindset, and behaviors, I believe you, too, will begin to see the importance of truly embracing these insights. Adopting these will help you deepen your faith in God and provide you with a perspective to bring you hope and inspiration as you battle cancer.

#1: Mindset
Cancer doesn't define you

The word *cancer* is intimidating, and naturally, if you are given this diagnosis, you may immediately assume you will die or your quality of life will be affected. Modern medicine, coupled with homeopathy treatments, is so advanced now that the probability of death for most cancers has decreased. However, there is always the chance death may occur.

My philosophy going into this health challenge was this: *I will fight until I can't fight any longer, and I will fight from strength, not as a victim or sickly person.* However, I was ready to accept death if that was the outcome God planned. I would try and enjoy the blessings all around me while I remained on this earth. Cancer would not define me, but it would show me how to approach life differently.

I struggle even today with calling myself a cancer survivor. I never felt comfortable giving the illness an identity; I felt that labeling it gave the disease a more prominent position in my life than it deserved. At first, understanding what I was facing and how it would be treated required discussing cancer in depth and by name, but once that treatment plan was in place, I was ready to move on from this label. I felt that calling myself a cancer survivor continued to give the illness visibility in my life. Cancer was a battle at a certain point in my life. It didn't define my past or my future, and I refused to let it drive my thoughts.

God reminds us in Exodus 13:3–8 about the importance of focusing on the right things. Moses, under God's direction and power, had helped the Israelites escape from bondage. Once they were free, God instructed them to remember to celebrate what he did for them. Focusing on and being thankful for what is holy, true, and good matters.

I find the way we look at cancer as a society interesting. We seem to elevate cancer in how we communicate about it. If someone has a heart attack, do we, for the rest of that person's life, refer to them as a heart attack survivor? For some reason, society keeps reminding us that cancer has survivors. Many diseases have survivors. I think our communication approach keeps the threat of cancer in our minds and creates fear, and I refuse to give cancer any more of my time than it already took. While some embrace being called a cancer survivor and overcoming obstacles, I prefer to talk about all the blessings this experience gave me. Cancer changed my life, not because I am a survivor, but because I became more open to what God wanted to show me.

God provided me with the wisdom to frame cancer in the right context. Consider for a moment the opportunity to reframe your perspective about cancer. Cancer is a health condition; it is not who you are. It can be a wake-up call to help you grow in your faith. Trials are often the only way God gets our attention because we are more open to embracing him at those times. Cancer is an opportunity to redefine your faith, and it can give you a new lens through which to look at the world. With this change in perspective, you may see, like I did, that cancer is the pathway to character growth and, as such, is a gift. God has a plan for your life that is better than what you can ever imagine. Don't allow cancer to define who you are or limit who you can be. Instead, allow your response to cancer be what defines you.

See Applying Insights in the Reflection & Action section to reflect more deeply on the insight that cancer doesn't define you.

#2: Character
Managing emotion grows character

No one can deny that getting a diagnosis of cancer is scary. You can expect to go through many emotions as you understand and begin to address your health challenges. The Elisabeth Kübler-Ross Change Curve Model highlights people's various reactions when faced with a significant change, including shock, denial, anger, bargaining, depression, and acceptance.[16] These emotional reactions are not necessarily sequential, and you may, in fact, experience many emotions at the same time. Allow yourself some grace in managing your emotions and let yourself, at the right time, move beyond the negative emotions to acceptance and action.

I find it interesting that one of the gifts God gave me as a business professional was the expertise in managing change. For decades, I have helped executives around the world manage systematic organizational change. This experience helped me deeply appreciate how each person may process and respond to situations differently and how managing emotions and behaviors are an important aspect of achieving a successful outcome. Because of this expertise, I suspect that I moved through the phases of change a little easier than someone who doesn't have this background. When I think of the connection between my professional and personal life, I can't help but smile with amazement and awe that, once again, God gave me the chance to develop talents that helped me both professionally and personally.

Let me take a moment to highlight a few details that illustrate how I was impacted emotionally through a few of these change phases.

For me, the shock phase was the most traumatic. Facing your own mortality changes your perspective. In retrospect, I should have had someone with me when I received the news that I had cancer—for support and to capture information since it was hard to concentrate on what the doctor was telling me after receiving such devastating news.

I was in shock for almost a month. I looked at the world differently as I observed people going about their regular tasks. Everyone seemed so carefree, so fortunate. I yearned to get back to those mundane tasks of normal life without the heavy burden of worrying about life and death.

I experienced frustration and anger along the way—more in the beginning as I became overwhelmed by all the information I had to absorb, numerous tests, and the myriad of doctors and appointments and decisions I had to make along the way.

I vividly remember one situation where I became angry with my husband while trying to schedule my chemo treatments. I wanted to have treatments on certain days and preferred mornings. My husband was granted time off work to take me to my appointments, but he also needed to minimize the impact of his absence on his job and coworkers. For him, being gone in the morning created more complications. He preferred to have the appointments scheduled later so he could work most of the day and leave work a little early.

I became frustrated with my husband because I felt, at that time, that he chose work over me, and I thought my treatment should be the highest priority. I told him in anger that I didn't need him to drive me and I would just take a taxi or the bus to and from the chemo appointments. Back in those days, ride-sharing services such as Uber and Lyft were not available. As I contemplated what to do next, I was anxious about finding my own way to my chemo treatments because I did not want to be unnecessarily exposed to germs since my immune system was compromised and would get weaker as I progressed in my chemo treatment. After much debate, I booked the appointments at the end of the day so my husband could drive me.

Looking back, I was clearly not objective. Stress caused me to become self-absorbed. At the time, I did not appreciate that he was trying to balance his work and employer needs with trying to care for me in the best way possible. It was never fair for me to question his intentions. It was a lesson in humility when I realized that when someone cannot help in the way you want or expect, it doesn't mean they are not supportive, but they may have other realistic demands that need to be addressed before they can help.

The other time I became frustrated was in communicating with my surgeon about procedure options. The surgeon was highly skilled and specialized in breast cancer, but her communication approach was not what I expected. Because I was still trying to understand the surgical options, I did extensive research and captured dozens of questions to ask the doctor during each visit. I'm one of those people who asks many questions to ensure I have a full understanding up-front, which can annoy some people who don't have the time or interest in answering tons of questions.

At each appointment, I would pull out my list of questions. After the second appointment, the doctor seemed annoyed with me and told me my questions would be answered in time by various doctors (not just her). I became so frustrated that I was being silenced and not heard at a time when I needed answers.

After the surgeon made her views known, I did not feel comfortable continuing with her as my doctor. I began to search for another surgeon who would actually listen to me. I scheduled time with my radiologist to ask for recommendations on other potential surgeons. The radiologist listened to me and shared his perspective, and his advice changed how I moved forward. You can read more about our conversation in Insight #7 entitled "Support: Resources are provided at the right time." However, in summary, I will say my frustration was diffused as a result of the radiologist's kindness and compassion.

What I didn't fully appreciate at the time was that the surgeon had just one role, and it was not to oversee the entire treatment plan to address my cancer. She was not the oncologist. The surgeon was, however, one of the first doctors I had to engage with since surgery was one of the first actions taken to remove the disease. The expectation that the surgeon would answer all my questions was, in fact, outside her scope and unreasonable. I just didn't realize it at the time. Level heads prevailed, and she remained my surgeon.

I was able to move through the negative change phases (shock, frustration, anger) and toward the acceptance phase fairly quickly, primarily because of the following reasons:

+ Some people question why they have to deal with a specific disease and believe it is unfair. This thought process reinforces a victim mentality and often spurs feelings of denial, anger, or depression. I chose to spend my time equipping myself for the battle rather than wasting time and energy on why I had to go through the fight.

+ Another talent I received from God was problem-solving. After the shock wore off, I approached cancer as a problem that was now defined and needed to be resolved. I put aside my emotions and focused on acquiring the data and information I needed to feel confident in the pathway forward. I spent many, many hours researching and gathering information to better understand what I was dealing with, and I looked at the problem from multiple lenses (life expectancy, probability of reoccurrence, speed at which the cancer was growing, quality of life, and treatment options, including traditional medicine and homeopathy). All this information was essential as I faced a multitude of decisions associated with my treatment plan. Looking at cancer as a problem that could be solved provided me with some level of control, which, in turn, helped me focus forward rather than dwell on what I could not change.

+ I was also blessed with an employer that had exceptional disability policies that allowed me to take disability leave from my job during my treatment and reduced the stress of having to juggle work while going through the various treatments. I continue to thank God for this. I have so much empathy for those who do not have this luxury and must continue to work while going through treatment. Because I did not have to worry about my job or finances, I could focus solely on my health and getting better.

Accept and acknowledge that you will experience various emotions, and give yourself grace when you have emotions that you may or may not expect. When you experience negative emotions, take a moment to reach out to God for support and guidance. Think about Proverbs 19:11 (GNT), which says, "If you are sensible, you will control your temper. When someone wrongs you, it is a great virtue to ignore it." Focus on what you can control and the goodness that is in you and around you. Changing your perspective will allow you to manage your emotions and grow in character.

I never prayed specifically for help in managing my emotions, nor did I understand at the time the connection between my emotions and my character. However, as I began to be more aware of my emotions, I changed the way I behaved (more patience, tolerance, and gratitude) and how I looked at situations. As I began to see the benefits of these changes, I began to transform. I was kinder and happier and had more self-control. I had more joy and peace in my life. What I didn't realize at the time was that the Spirit of God was transforming my character by helping me address those areas where I was emotionally weak.

See Applying Insights in the Reflection & Action section to reflect more deeply on the insight that managing emotion grows character.

#3: Faith
I am not alone

God does not want you to be alone. He wants you to forge strong relationships with him and others to help you navigate life's challenges and triumphs. This is reinforced in Matthew 22:37–39 (GNT), where Jesus declared, "'Love the Lord your God with all your heart, with all your soul, and with all your mind'" and that we should "'Love your neighbor as you love yourself.'" In Revelation 3:20 (NIV), Jesus reinforces the importance of a relationship with him when he says, "Here I am! I stand at the door and knock. If anyone hears my voice and opens the door, I will come in and eat with that person, and they with me."

When you are faced with severe health challenges, it is easy to become isolated. Isolation could be self-imposed or caused by others, such as people avoiding you because they don't know what to say. Nurturing close relationships is necessary for both physical and mental health and is key to avoiding being alone.

Because of my introverted tendencies and the amount of energy that went into battling cancer, interacting with others was not always a top priority for me. In some ways, I was perfectly fine with having no calls or visitors. Like most introverts, I become drained in social settings. For me, feeling isolated was never an issue, as I felt the love and support of my family in various ways, including prayers, cards, calls, and visits. I also had a deep faith that God was with me every step of the way.

Through God's grace, I grew to expand my perspective and embrace a broader community, including strangers. I mentioned earlier that I wore my baldness with pride. This visual display would often trigger reactions in others. Strangers would stop me while I was shopping to give me words of encouragement, give me a hug, or share their stories. My baldness impacted others differently. In every case, it triggered a deeply emotional reaction based on an event in the individual's life.

While I was going through treatment, it was critical for me to be mindful of being exposed to germs, as my immune system was in overdrive fighting cancer and trying to heal itself. I did not want a stranger touching or getting close to me, but the compassion these people showed touched my heart time and time again. I began to realize these interactions not only helped me but also the individual who took the time to stop and show genuine care, concern, and hope. This was a key takeaway as I began to become more aware of how my situation or presence impacted other people. I could affect people in a positive way if I moved beyond myself and began to appreciate those around me more fully.

A deep faith in God and his plan for my life also gave me the confidence to know I was not alone. This entire book is about all the blessings that were bestowed on me and the active and visible signs God used to show me he was with me the whole time I was battling cancer. I love the poem entitled "Footprints,"[17] which highlights how God will walk beside you in life but will also pick you up and carry you when you need it most. With this kind of love and support, how could I feel lonely? A key way to feel that connection with God was through daily prayer.

Although you may be blessed to have friends or family in your life to help you through your journey, leverage these relationships fully to remind yourself that you are not alone. Look more broadly and through your daily dealing with others, and you may find a deeper connection that can provide you with community, inspiration, and hope. Also, do not let one more day pass without making a commitment to nurture a relationship with God. God is all-powerful, and you will never be alone if you have faith in him and allow him to help you with what he knows you need. Isaiah 41:10 (NLT) reminds you that God will always be with you: "Don't be afraid, for I am with you. / Don't be discouraged, for I am your God. / I will strengthen you and help you."

See Applying Insights in the Reflection & Action section to reflect more deeply on the insight that you are not alone.

#4: Empathy
Caring for others brings joy

As I confronted my new reality and what I had to deal with after my cancer diagnosis, my view of the world changed and became narrower. I found myself not having the capacity to care about anyone besides myself. All my energy was focused on battling cancer and getting well. My priorities were very clear in my mind. However, as I progressed in my journey, I started to have a deeper respect for the struggles of those around me, and this led to my priorities shifting.

When people looked at me, they did not know the internal challenges I was going through, as my health issues were not visible early on. Before losing my hair, only those closest to me knew my struggles. Later, when I became bald, it was not inconceivable that strangers would conclude I had a health issue.

I began to think about how people might be struggling in ways I could not see. I put a higher level of importance on my interactions with others. I started to respond differently in my day-to-day engagements. I was kinder and more empathetic. For example, when I was cut off by another driver on the road, someone provided me with poor service, or I had to wait longer than expected, I no longer became angry or frustrated. I would instead remind myself that I had no idea what hurt or circumstance might be behind the situation. Instead of responding with negative emotions, I began to respond with empathy and concern.

Time took on a new meaning. I was less rushed and began to appreciate every moment, every interaction. With the demands of life, it is easy to pass people with a quick hello but never really know them or what they are going through. God began to reshape how I looked at others. This new perspective, once again, didn't come about because I asked for this in prayer, but it was a gift God showed me as he artfully opened my eyes to what I was missing when I focused on the wrong priorities. This broader lesson is described in Luke 10:40–41, which tells how Mary focused rightfully on God while her sister Martha was distracted by tasks.

I began to spend more quality time with people I knew, which not only provided me with support but also gave me the opportunity to get to know these individuals at a much deeper level. It created moments for me to encourage others rather than being solely focused on myself. I found by taking a little time to connect with people, I learned so much about what was really going on in their lives and what difficulties they had. There was a new purpose forming in my life that was not about me but about how I could support others. It brings me such joy when I am given an opportunity to help others.

Today, my daily prayer list is quite long, as I pray for all my family and friends who are going through various challenges, which I only grew to understand after making a conscious effort to spend time with each individual and to nurture these cherished relationships. I was given a true gift when I could be there to help someone else when they needed it even while I was battling cancer. Through these interactions, I had a deeper awareness of how much people need each other.

Life gives all of us challenges. No one can escape hardship, as we live in a fallen world. As I began to see people through a lens of empathy, I realized I would never know the drivers behind the actions of others. I found that grace and kindness went a long way in how I responded to the bad behaviors of others and reduced my negative responses to specific circumstances. Kindness truly de-escalates a situation. I became less self-centered and self-absorbed as I spent more time listening and helping others.

Being more empathetic and caring about others strengthened my relationships, changed my point of view, grew my character, and brought more compassion to my life. This also was an example of God knowing exactly what I needed. He showed me I was surrounded by people who could help me and who also needed my help.

Although you may be overwhelmed by your situation, consider opening your heart and reaching out to those who may need you. Philippians 2:4 (GNT) reminds us to "look out for one another's interests, not just for your own." This may be hard to do when difficulties are distracting you. The simple gesture of caring for others and putting your own interests aside for a moment can bring you joy and many benefits you don't even realize you need.

See Applying Insights in the Reflection & Action section to reflect more deeply on the insight that caring for others brings joy.

#5: Petition
Prayer is powerful and comforting

As you face your health challenge, you will have a myriad of emotions. At times, you will feel powerless and need comfort. Other times, you may feel tired and sad. It can be overwhelming when you are faced with the complexity of any disease, confusion over all the terminology and information, and uncertainty regarding how to proceed. It could feel like your world is spinning out of control and there is no hope. Whether or not you are a spiritual person, there are times when you know you need help. God is waiting to help you if you just ask. He loves you dearly and can bring you comfort and hope. He may use various methods to show you his love, including through his words reflected in the Bible, music, prayer, and other people.

Before my cancer, I believed in God and prayed periodically. I was brought up in the Catholic faith and was baptized and confirmed in the church. Although I spent decades in the Catholic Church, I never really felt a strong connection to the church institution. I guess you can say I was more spiritual than religious. I also felt the Catholic Church did a poor job of engaging with the community to help them better understand the faith. I found the Catholic environment focused more on rules, rituals, and condemnation rather than on creating an environment that was welcoming for those who were not perfect (and that would be all of us).

After the Catholic child abuse scandal that rocked the worldwide church, I found it harder and harder to embrace the traditions that felt unimportant and unauthentic. At the time, there was a conservative pope who was making changes to numerous rituals performed during the church Mass, including changes to how parishioners responded to certain passages. I struggled with the church's priorities, given the lack of accountability and tangible action related to the child abuse scandal and the increased focus on changing Mass protocols. I felt the Catholic Church had clearly lost its way. I could not ignore the inaction of the leadership at that time in supporting the victims and addressing the issues immediately. I could not, in good conscience, follow leaders who acted like this. Although I no longer consider myself a Catholic, I continue to have the utmost respect for my brothers and sisters in Christ who find inspiration, faith, and hope in the Catholic Church. We are all part of God's family, and we must not forget that.

Despite my struggle with the Catholic institution, I never lost my connection to God. Previously, God was present in some of my early challenges, and I knew that with faith, he could do wonders in my life. So, when I got cancer, I naturally relied on prayer for comfort and asked for guidance. I surrounded myself with positive and encouraging words whenever possible.

Every day, I listened to the Christian radio station K-LOVE.[18] So many of the songs comforted me and gave me inspiration and hope. The music felt nourishing and created a positive environment for me. Many of the songs reminded me of God's glory, highlighted the struggles or challenges of others so I knew I was not alone, and emphasized the importance of faith. These songs were prayers set to music. Music helped me transcend into another place. It made me aware of how grateful I was that God was reaching me through these lyrical prayers. Music nourished my soul every day.

I also asked my family to pray for me. At that time, I joked that many of my siblings were much better Christians than I was. I felt like I was in good hands since I was confident God listened to their prayers, even if he wasn't going to listen to mine, given my struggle with the Catholic faith. I knew I was blessed with a family that believed in Christ, and in my heart I knew it was essential that I surround myself with their love and support during my journey. According to James 5:16 (GNT), "The prayer of a good person has a powerful effect." It reminded me how fortunate I was to have an entire family of believers who could help me through my journey by petitioning God for my health.

One blessing God showed me is the power of collective prayer. As soon as my family started praying, I felt different. It is hard to describe the impact of this. I felt the prayers just lifted me up, and I had so much hope. While I had some doubt about my own petitions, I had absolute faith in my family members' abilities to approach God on my behalf. I felt surrounded by love the entire time I was battling cancer. This love was visible in my family interactions and prayers, and I truly felt God was present to help me through the challenges that each day brought. There is no doubt in my mind that collective or group prayer was instrumental in providing the support and comfort I needed each step of the way.

When I prayed during my cancer battle, I prayed that I would live. However, I recognized that I did not know the outcome and I could possibly die. Although I chose to focus my prayers on living, I also accepted that it may be God's will that it was my time to be with God in heaven. I was reminded of when Jesus said, "Father, if you are willing, please take this cup of suffering away from me. Yet I want your will to be done, not mine" (Luke 22:42 NLT). If it was my time to die, I would make every minute count and live my remaining days in a way that pleased God and aligned with his plans for my life.

Like any relationship, your relationship with God must be nurtured. He wants you to glorify him, share your struggles, and lean on him for support. In turn, he has many blessings available to you. I made— and still make—God a priority by spending time with him in prayer and reflection every day. I talk to God from the heart rather than saying the same prayers over and over. This was so different for me since growing up in the Catholic faith was more about reading and repeating the same prayers. Matthew

6:7 (NLT) says, "When you pray, don't babble on and on as the Gentiles do. They think their prayers are answered merely by repeating their words again and again." I have found prayer to be much more powerful when you speak to God directly as your heavenly father rather than a distant figure you don't know. As a father, he wants to hear what is in your heart.

For those who are new to prayer or just want a refresher, read Matthew 6:5–15, which shows us how to think about and structure our prayer time. Prayer is an opportunity for us to be alone with God and just talk to him.

In addition to dedicating time for prayer each day, I would pause for brief prayer moments as I noticed beautiful imagery around me that made me smile. It was amazing how taking short pauses during the day to be grateful brought me comfort and joy by recognizing and feeling the goodness of God. His presence is all around you; you just need to be open to seeing it.

One pastor mentioned that when you pray, be specific which will make it easier for you to recognize when your prayers have been answered. I now have a running list of all the prayers God has answered, which reminds me every day about his power and the direct and active involvement he has in my life. When prayers are not answered, I keep petitioning. Unanswered prayers do not mean God doesn't listen. He knows what you need and when you need it. Always remember God's time is different than your time, and his timing is always perfect.

Individual and collective prayers can have a positive effect on your cancer journey. Reach out to your church, family, and friends and ask them to pray for you. Ask them to pray for specific areas you are struggling with throughout your journey, such as a surgery decision, emotional support, competent doctors, and finances. If you don't know anyone who can pray for you, another option is to send prayer requests via the K-LOVE prayer line (at the time of publication, the phone number is 800-525-5683) or their website (klove.com/ministry/prayer).

Prayer will bring you comfort and hope as you anticipate what God will do in your life and the lives of others who are helping you through your journey. Open your eyes to his goodness by developing a relationship with him and having faith in his plan. Prayer is our conduit to God, and it strengthens our bond with him. God has a larger, more profound purpose for my life and your life. Allow him to show you what that is.

See Applying Insights in the Reflection & Action section to reflect more deeply on the insight that prayer is powerful and comforting.

#6: Guidance
God speaks to us in many ways

You may be wondering how you know if God is listening. How does he communicate his will in your life? Throughout my life, God has shown his presence. Each time I received a message or blessing from God, it changed me significantly. God often makes himself visible in our darkest times. This is because we are more open to hearing from him when we need help. In good times, people take pride in their own abilities and often think the sole reason for success is themselves and their hard work. I, too, had this perspective at the beginning of my cancer journey. This belief couldn't be further from the truth, as God is the one who gives us the talents and resources to succeed.

God has shown himself to me in various ways. I often think of the verse in John 20:29 (NLT) that says, "You believe because you have seen me. Blessed are those who believe without seeing me." I have seen the power of God in my life through the mini miracles he has blessed me with. I have so much gratitude for receiving a small glimpse of what God is capable of and for feeling that he loves me so much that he made his presence known in various ways. I praise those who have not had these experiences yet still believe. These are people who demonstrate true faith.

God has shown himself to me in both good and challenging times. However, to illustrate how God actually showed up, I'll focus on the challenging times given the situation you are facing.

Years ago, my former company was laying off workers. I had a supervisor who I felt at the time was just wicked and lacked a moral compass. In her quest to please her manager, she chose to participate in an attack on my character with the intent of sabotaging my career while covering up the egregious behavior of one of my team members, who I will call "Sally."

Sally had a personal relationship with my supervisor's manager and was a poor performer. From my perspective, it seemed Sally did not like being held accountable for her work and used her relationship with my supervisor's manager to try to discredit me after I gave her a poor performance rating. One day, out of the blue, I was summoned to a meeting with my supervisor and her manager. While my supervisor sat silent, the manager verbally assaulted my reputation and said I was a poor leader.

My supervisor wanted to be promoted, so rather than objectively evaluating the situation, she went along with whatever her manager said. I knew in my heart that the manager's view was influenced by Sally and his relationship with her. I felt crushed and defeated after working so hard to build a competent and high-performing team.

The situation was extremely difficult to navigate. Although Sally's claims about me were untrue, management was not interested in gathering the facts to assess the appropriate course of action. I felt repeatedly attacked and persecuted for doing my job. I thought I had no support or anyone I could turn to.

I am someone who believes strongly in integrity, so the attack on my character without the ability to defend myself was especially hurtful. After months of trying to resolve the situation and trusting that good would prevail over evil or facts over fiction, I was given notice that I was being laid off. I was thankful the company had a separation policy that allowed me six months to try and find another job within the company before being laid off.

Losing my job, in addition to the personal conflicts caused by the work environment, was extremely stressful. To get away from the situation, I took a temporary role in another city with the same company, and I felt the person who offered me a temporary job was an angel who saved me. Having some distance between me and those who were trying to hurt me felt like a lifeline.

During the long commute to my temporary job, I experienced a lot of pain while sitting. I eventually saw a doctor who conducted X-rays and determined I had a crack in my tailbone that was causing the pain. That meant I was facing physical pain as well as emotional pain, but my situation became even worse.

I learned a short time later that I was pregnant and became concerned that I had exposed my unborn child to radiation since the recent tailbone X-rays were around my pelvic region. My life became a nightmare as I worried constantly that I may have hurt the baby in my womb. I tried and tried to get the doctor to tell me about the level of radiation I had been exposed to so I could seek proper medical guidance. The doctor did not cooperate nor provide any information on the level of radiation exposure; I assume because of legal concerns. The lack of control and the thought of what type of damage I may have unknowingly caused my child was terrifying. I was under considerable stress and felt my life was spinning out of control.

I was devastated and had many, many days and nights when I spent hours crying and praying. I felt my world was collapsing around me, and it was all triggered by circumstances I could not control or resolve on my own. The potential lack of a job became less important as I faced growing concerns about the health of my unborn child. It was hard for me to function every day, and I saw no way out of the place I was in.

God heard my prayers. Isaiah 35:4 (NIV) says "Be strong, do not fear; / your God will come, / he will come with vengeance," and he truly showed up in force. One evening, I was flipping through TV channels and stopped on a religious channel when I heard someone singing a beautiful song. I had never heard the song before. I listened to the entire song; it moved me deeply as it was angelic and pure. After it was done, I continued flipping the channels, not really thinking much of it.

I went to work the next day, and I was listening to my radio, which I did every day. Typically, the station I listened to played soul and rap music. I was feeling especially sad on this day. At some point in the morning, I was surprised when that beautiful song I had heard on the TV the previous night blared through my radio. I sat there in shock and awe. How could that song be playing on the soul/rap station? I was confused for a moment and then noticed my radio had fallen on its side. I suddenly felt the full force and power of God's love. Immediately, all the stresses left my body. I felt the weight of those burdens disappear. I cried in sheer amazement and awe as I felt God's presence. He had been there with me all along. Peace and love swept over me.

The same day the music came through my radio, I received a call offering me a permanent job in another part of the company, which meant I would not be laid off. I also received a call from a company doctor who reassured me there was a low probability the radiation would have harmed my child. Months later, my daughter was born with no negative impacts from the X-rays.

I was elated that my concerns about my daughter were unfounded and that I was once again employed. This was more than I could have asked for, but God wasn't done. The job I took became the catalyst for a three-grade promotion a year later, which was unheard of in my company at that time. I often think about Genesis 50:20 (NIV), which says, "You intended to harm me, but God intended it for good to accomplish what is now being done." I let go of all the negative feelings about what led to these events and focused on how God turned something bad into something good.

I experienced a miracle when God lifted the burdens from me and then created a sequence of events to reassure me of what he wanted to do in my life. To this day, when I think about this miracle, I stand in awe of God and feel truly blessed to have seen and felt his mercy and grace. God was there for me like no one else could be. Once you experience this kind of love and power, it can't help but change you forever.

I used the prior story to illustrate various ways God spoke to me before I had cancer, as it is such a vivid example of his presence. While battling cancer, I felt God's nearness as a result of collective prayer and inspiring messages I heard on K-LOVE. As I listened to the station, people would call in and talk about how God had changed their lives, which gave me hope. So many times, a song or a person spoke words that were exactly what I needed to hear. I found when I removed the world's distractions and instead opened myself up to what God wanted me to hear, I felt his closeness and was inspired. A third key way God showed his presence was when I returned to work after completing my treatment plan. I describe in detail what transpired in Insight #10, "Seeing goodness in others is transformative."

Recently, while addressing a different challenge, I felt it was God's desire for me to tell the truth and address a deeply held family secret. I—and all those involved—prayed a lot about this. We often talked as a family, and I reached out to a pastor to confirm the best course of action. I felt confident in the plan, but there were others who were not as sure about the approach and did not want to proceed.

While I was trying to get alignment on the plan, a little pink book called *365 Encouraging Verses of the Bible for Women*[19] fell off my bookshelf. I couldn't remember the last time I read this book, and there was no reason why it should have fallen. It was surrounded by lots of other books. I didn't give it a second thought and placed the book back on the shelf. A little while later, the book was on the floor again. It made me smile as I knew God was trying to send me a message. I opened the book to the page that was flagged. The verse was Deuteronomy 31:6 (NIV), which says, "Be strong and courageous. Do not be afraid or terrified because of them, for the Lord your God goes with you; he will never leave you nor forsake you."

I felt God was reminding me that our plan was actually his plan. God wanted me to move forward, and he was with us. He was also working through the hearts of all those involved to ensure a positive outcome. The plan was executed, and the results were better than anyone could have hoped for. This was a great reminder that when your plans are aligned with God's plans, amazing things can happen.

I cherish these moments when God has shown me his presence. I am humbled by them because I feel that I am unworthy to receive such gifts. It does bring me great joy that I have him in my corner and that, no matter what happens, he will always be there for me.

Here are a few ways God may choose to speak to you if you are open to hearing from him:

His Word: God often speaks to us through his Word or the Scriptures in the Bible. Have you ever noticed the same concept or words keep showing up? Did you read a verse that was exactly what you needed to hear? When people read the Bible, they take away different messages because God talks to each one of us based on what we need. If you are not reading the Bible, you are missing out on a key way God may talk to you.

Holy Spirit: The Holy Spirit is the Spirit of God who lives in all those who believe in him. The Holy Spirit is like a trusted coach and advocate who has the instructional manual to life to help you through life's challenges. The Holy Spirit educates by revealing God's truth at the right time when you need it. If you are open to receiving his message, the Holy Spirit will plant ideas and thoughts in your mind and suggest specific steps that align with God's plans for your life. Psalm 32:8 (GNT) says, "I will teach you the way you should go; / I will instruct you and advise you." You always have a choice to follow his guidance or not. However, when you do obey, you will begin to see positive changes taking place in your life. It is through this process of listening, reflecting, praying, and taking action that you will transform.

Prayer: Have you ever felt God's presence while you are praying or realized the benefits of prayer, such as a feeling of forgiveness or a burden being lifted? Prayer is a direct line of communication to God. If you are not praying, you are not utilizing an essential channel to understand God's will for your life and to receive his blessings.

People: God talks to us through other people. Have you ever struggled with an issue, and then a person happens to make a comment that helps you with that worry? That could be God trying to reach you. While writing this book, several times, one of my pastors shared a message that was similar to what I was writing. I believe this was God's way of telling me I was on the right track.

His Works: During my cancer journey, I embraced the healing power of nature. God created a beautiful environment, and when I embraced this beauty, I felt God's proximity. I used to take walks every day and reflect on the natural blessings God has provided. I would walk on grass and just enjoy what it felt like on my feet. I would look at the hills, the sky, and the birds with gratitude. I was fortunate to live in a place with a lot of open space, and I took advantage of being outside as much as possible. I thought it gave me a chance to glorify God and to feel his awesomeness for creating such beauty that also heals the soul.

Visions: Many Scriptures highlight how God sent messages through dreams. For example, in Matthew 2:12, God warned the Magi in a dream to return to their country by a different road than they originally planned to ensure their safety. Dreams are hard to interpret, and most of us are not prophets who have a gift from God about how to interpret them. Leviticus 19:31 reminds us *not* to consult mediums, so if you have a dream, look to the Bible and Scripture experts to help you determine what the dream might mean.

Roadblocks: God may create roadblocks if you are going down the wrong path or if you need to learn a lesson before taking the next step. Just like your earthly father, God corrects his children out of love, as mentioned in Hebrews 12:6. As you face roadblocks, keep in mind that God is more concerned with your character than he is with material items. Maybe God is not closing a door but delaying it because you need to learn a lesson or events beyond your control need to happen before you can be successful. When your plans are aligned with God's plans for your life, you will see amazing doors open.

As you deepen your relationship with God, you will begin to see how he is actively working in your life. Be open to how messages may be coming to you, and look for ways he may be giving you a message to help you in your life's journey. Ask God for help to receive his words, and glorify him when you do. Slow down and give yourself the time and space to hear from him.

See Applying Insights in the Reflection & Action section to reflect more deeply on the insight that God speaks to us in many ways.

#7: Support Resources are provided at the right time

When you are faced with a major illness, you may be affected emotionally, spiritually, financially, physically, socially, and relationally. These changes may impact you all at once or at different times throughout your journey. You have a lot to think about as you try to address the various dimensions of your cancer journey. Your frustration may increase when you don't have the information you need or don't know how to proceed. However, I found that God provided the right resources to me at the right time.

When I first learned about my cancer diagnosis, I was faced with understanding my treatment options while trying to comprehend the short- and long-term disability policies of my state and employer. I was fortunate to work in a state that gave me time off with full pay for about eight weeks. I also thanked God for my employer, which had policies that did not require me to work while going through treatment. I was off work for about eight months, which covered time for preparation, surgery, chemo, and radiation.

As I was deciding about treatment options, I was offered the opportunity to participate in genetic testing. I welcomed the testing, as it was a critical piece of information to use in determining which surgery option I would pursue. God presented this option at the right time and before I needed to make the surgical decision.

The last area relating to the treatment plan was in the selection of doctors. I previously mentioned that I was assigned a surgeon who was very skilled, but she did not address my concerns in a way that made me feel heard. I thought I needed to find another surgeon but was talked out of it by the radiation oncology doctor. He was patient and reinforced the importance of skill when choosing a surgeon. He reminded me that once the surgery was done, I did not need to interact with the surgeon any longer. He repeated that the surgeon I was assigned was an exceptional surgeon. This discussion changed my perspective. I felt truly heard, and he influenced my thinking by listening and providing a viewpoint I needed to hear. I truly believe it was God once again giving me resources and insights at the right time. I stayed with the surgeon, and she was excellent. I had no complications, and aesthetically, the scar was very small considering the type of surgery I had.

Other resources God blessed me with during treatment included an oncologist who was highly skilled and caring; help from family and friends, whether it be kind words, prayers, a cooked meal, or a listening ear; a nutritionist to ensure I was eating the right foods; various books and research to give me strategies and actions to aid in my recovery; classes to interact with others going through similar challenges to give me support; and wigs to help me deal with my hair loss.

My supervisor, Jane, was also another resource. To this day, I am so deeply touched by how she handled my leave and my return to work. She visited me on her own time to see how I was doing throughout my treatments. Jane called me periodically to give support and to reinforce that it was all right to focus on myself and not worry about work at all. She also demonstrated a deep understanding of what I needed when I returned to work.

After my treatment ended, I had what is commonly referred to as *chemo brain*. According to the National Cancer Institute, chemo brain is a term used to describe a cancer patient's thinking or memory issues.[20] I was not prepared for this side effect; I hadn't seen any signs during treatment and had not done any research on it.

When I was cleared to go back to work, my brain didn't function as it had before. I had a difficult time concentrating and remembering people and their names. I couldn't connect or make sense of basic concepts. I had a hard time analyzing information. I used to have so much pride in my ability to solve complex problems, but that talent seemed to disappear. I tried to give myself grace when I couldn't remember details and reminded myself that it wasn't my fault so I should not feel bad or embarrassed about my memory struggles.

My brain felt different like there was a lot of misfiring happening. My thoughts were there but were disparate and not connected in a coherent or meaningful way. It gave me a glimpse into how fragile life is. I felt sad at times, knowing that my mind might never work in the same way as it did prior to chemo.

God gives us our talents, but those talents can be easily taken, and I was given the gift to see how life would be without some of my abilities. This is why it is so important for me today to praise God for the talents I have; it is through his true grace that I have regained them and can use them in a way that pleases him. I am reminded of 2 Corinthians 3:5 (NLT), which reinforces that God is the source of our talent: "It is not that we think we are qualified to do anything on our own. Our qualification comes from God." It is a true gift that I now know what life would be like if I didn't have the same capabilities.

I never told my supervisor about my chemo brain, as I did not want to appear like I couldn't do my job. Although we never discussed it, Jane somehow knew I needed to slowly transition into my work. She assigned me a special project so I wouldn't become overwhelmed with managing the full scope of my job. My work seemed to take much longer, and simple tasks were much more difficult to do. She allowed me to move back to the workplace in a way that helped me feel accomplished and stay positive. After I completed the project, she was gracious in celebrating this key milestone and slowly introduced more work as I regained my capabilities. Although I was able to handle the full job within a few months, it took about one and a half years to feel confident that my brain was working correctly and firing on all cylinders again.

I'm not sure how successful I would have been at work if I had not been blessed with the supervisor I had. Jane modeled all the fruit of the Spirit mentioned in Galatians 5:22–23 (GNT): "love, joy, peace, patience, kindness, goodness, faithfulness, humility, and self-control." It was not surprising that she eventually left the company to become a pastor. She was filled with God's Spirit, and through her, I was blessed.

God is a loving father. He will not only provide resources at the right time, but he will also provide resources you may not know you need, which was the case with my former supervisor Jane.

See Applying Insights in the Reflection & Action section to reflect more deeply on the insight that resources are provided at the right time.

#8: Forgiveness
Grace gives us the power to forgive

As you face the truth of your condition and search for information and support, it is easy to become self-centered. Your world, in some ways, will become narrower and in other ways, so much more complex while you are battling cancer. As you accept your new reality, you can expect to become intensely focused on you and what you need to do to make the right decisions about your treatment. It will be easy to become irritated or angry with others who do not act in a way you expect or who may bother you when you just want to be left alone because you are not feeling well. You also may become frustrated with yourself if you fail to meet your own expectations.

One of God's gifts to you during this life challenge is to provide you with people who can support you in unique ways. How you interact with others during this time can uplift your spirit or cause sadness and hurt in your relationships. I encourage you to think about how your illness is impacting others. This requires deeper self-awareness so you can respond in grace when others do not behave as you expect.

People respond differently when someone they know or care about has been diagnosed with an illness. One gift God gave me was realizing that my cancer journey was not all about me, and I needed to forgive anyone who did not behave as expected. Most people want to help, but they often don't know how and don't know what to say.

Initially, I was surprised at the different responses of family and friends. Some reacted as you would expect, and others did not. Many brought food; sent cards and flowers, books and stuffed animals; or stopped by to visit throughout the treatments. My oldest daughter offered to take a break from her college program to come home and care for me. My sister and her husband, who lived in a different state, took time away from their family and work to care for me while I was going through chemo. I was continuously reminded I was loved and cared for by my family and friends who found a variety of ways to show their support and compassion.

In addition, some close family and friends distanced themselves. At first, I was hurt by some of the reactions; however, as time progressed, I began to realize I was not the center of their worlds. People had busy, complex lives with their own challenges, and it was critical that I not judge but instead recognize that the world didn't revolve around me.

One individual sent me a book about positive thinking and included a personal note. At the time, I thought the note seemed to imply that I caused my cancer through negative thinking. I was hurt and couldn't imagine anyone making this type of comment to someone battling cancer. It is true that negative thinking can have a negative impact on your health, but blaming someone for cancer is hurtful, unnecessary, and not appropriate.

However, this situation highlights how easily gestures can be misinterpreted. Upon reflection, I now believe the individual was providing me with tools she felt were essential in managing my health over the long term. With a heart of forgiveness, you may find deeper meaning in situations when an individual initially disappoints or hurts you. Believe that people have good intentions, and accept gestures of kindness with gratitude and forgiveness rather than judgment.

I never had a conversation with the individuals who acted in ways I did not initially expect because I did not want them to carry the burden of regret, which is not healthy for the individuals or the relationships. I just imagined the myriad of responsibilities that may have caused the individuals to not reach out. It is an interesting exercise to think of possible reasons for inaction. For example, maybe the individual was going through their own crisis and did not want to burden me with it when they knew I needed to focus on myself. Maybe they did not know what to say, which made them uncomfortable, or they did not want to see me in a weakened state but instead wanted to think of me when I was healthy. Perhaps they were doing what they thought was the most helpful, such as praying for me every day, and I just didn't know it.

One regret on the topic of forgiveness had to do with my youngest daughter. My daughter was getting in trouble at school. It was a stressful time for our family, and she was quite rebellious. Many parents who have teenagers may understand the stress it creates when your child's path is going in the wrong direction. When I was diagnosed with cancer, my daughter was attending a Catholic school and was consistently breaking minor rules. She had so many infractions (related to lateness and clothing) that the school informed us they were expelling her. I pleaded with the school to allow her to stay and asked for assistance from our priest to advocate. We evaluated other schooling options and could not find an acceptable solution given the limited time she had before graduation. This situation caused me considerable stress at a time when I wanted to focus on my treatment. I felt distraught. I resented my daughter for only caring about herself and creating such conflict that I didn't need. I became angry and frustrated with her, as she didn't appear to care about her schooling situation or my illness. Early on, I thought it was strange that when we learned about my cancer diagnosis, she had no reaction. She basically acted as if nothing had changed. She never asked questions or acted concerned.

Although we convinced the school to keep her enrolled, her antics continued. I could not understand how anyone could treat a loved one in this way, given the severity of what I was going through. In anger, I made hurtful comments to her, and not surprisingly, she continued to act up. I blamed her for my situation. I told her that all the stress I had been under over the last few years in dealing with all her issues had impacted my health and caused me to get sick.

Years later, we talked about why she distanced herself, and she said it was because I had blamed her. It broke my heart. My precious daughter lived with the burden that she caused my cancer because I told her she had. This was a burden that I unfairly placed on her because I said hurtful words in anger that were fundamentally untrue.

I asked for her forgiveness and told her I did not believe she had caused my cancer and that it was said out of frustration and anger. I explained to her that stress is managed internally. No one can blame another person for how they respond to stress. If my daughter and I had had better coping skills, we would have handled all the stress associated with her high school years and my cancer very differently. I can never take back the hurtful words, and to this day, I deeply regret that I used words to hurt her. I placed a burden on her that she was not supposed to carry. Although I believe she has forgiven me, I am still working on forgiving myself for causing her pain when she was already going through so much. One of my biggest regrets is that I did not embrace the intent of Ephesians 4:29 (GNT): "Do not use harmful words, but only helpful words, the kind that build up and provide what is needed, so that what you say will do good to those who hear you." My words were hurtful and inexcusable.

Your cancer journey will impact your relationships. You may not know why people behave the way they do. You don't know what others are going through or how your illness may be affecting them. Be mindful to not say words that you will regret that could have lasting implications on the people you love. Showing grace means you forgive mistakes, lapses in judgment, and hurtful behaviors because no one is perfect. Accept whatever kindness you are given with gratitude, and assume people have good intentions so you can respond with grace and humility.

Lastly, learn to forgive yourself for actions you may have taken that hurt others. If there is an opportunity to ask for forgiveness, please do so. It is through grace that forgiveness can occur, even when you think you are not worthy.

See Applying Insights in the Reflection & Action section to reflect more deeply on the insight that grace gives us the power to forgive.

#9: Gratitude
Humility changes how we view life

Cancer has a way of changing your perspective by showing you what is important and what is not. All the possessions you wanted, all the accolades you received, all the events you experienced, and how you look don't matter when you are faced with life or death.

Prior to battling cancer, I was blessed with a wonderful family and a good job, and we were comfortable financially, which allowed us to travel and have unique experiences. My husband and I worked hard for decades and took time to enjoy the benefits of our efforts. Our family felt blessed to have the opportunity to travel and learn about diverse cultures.

I was especially driven from a career standpoint since I was raised in a family that reinforced the importance of work in achieving one's goals. If you wanted to get ahead, you had to work for it. I was employed by the same oil and gas company for much of my adult life, starting in an administrative capacity and working my way up through the management ranks. I had a strong work ethic, and at times, I worked ninety-hour weeks. I had so much pride and confidence in my ability to produce that it resulted in me not fully appreciating my impact on others. Some may have referred to me as a perfectionist. Delivering quality work was essential to me and, at times, came at the cost of my work/life balance. My standards have always been high, and I pushed others to achieve more than they thought possible. I felt pride when my team members would tell me they had never learned so much in any job before.

The intensity of delivering results year after year, began to change me. I found myself becoming more and more judgmental of how I looked at others and their approach to work. I was a constant overachiever who was thoroughly exhausted trying to maintain an arbitrary standard that only I cared about.

During a time when I was extremely burned out, I asked for God's help to make me more humble in order to change my expectations of myself and others. Humble people are aware of their shortcomings. They are not prideful, arrogant, or vain. After dedicating time to pray about humility, I was diagnosed with cancer. I am not suggesting that God gave me cancer so I could develop humility, but he did use my cancer battle to make me more humble.

While battling cancer, I had to learn to let go. I could not control the uncontrollable. I could not rely solely on my talents but had to rely on the talents and support of others. All the accomplishments I had thought were so necessary—exceeding expectations, amassing wealth, achieving accolades—no longer mattered.

One way cancer made me more humble was through my hair loss due to chemo. For women, this is especially hard. Going out without hair can be embarrassing for some. Many support groups offer wigs, scarves, and hats to reduce the social stigma associated with female baldness. I found that breaking the stereotype that women should not show their bare heads created opportunities to learn and laugh and appreciate life in a new way. For example, I realized I didn't need to use shampoo any longer. This had never occurred to me. It was just weird after spending so much money on shampoos and conditioners to no longer need them. I saved money by not purchasing these products and saved time when it came to showering and getting ready. A silver lining emerged. Instead of focusing on the negatives of baldness, I let cancer show me the benefits of baldness.

When I took a trip with my family to Yosemite, I realized how much our hair insulates our heads. My head was freezing, so I purchased a beanie at the local store. I had never once thought about the role of hair in holding in heat. Now, I have a new appreciation when I observe people with no hair. I assume they must have a hat close by.

When my hair started to grow again, I would look in the mirror and just laugh. I had those little baby hairs that would blow in the wind. I joked that I felt like a baby ostrich with fine puffs of hair moving in the breeze. I got sheer enjoyment from an idea so basic and silly.

Another lesson I learned regarding humility is that what God gives us, he can also take away in an instant (see Job 1:21). For all those years I prided myself on using my abilities to achieve success, I never appreciated that all my gifts came from God. I should have been thanking God for the talents he gave me rather than thinking all my triumphs came from me. I was prideful and arrogant.

I mentioned earlier that after I finished chemo, I experienced chemo brain, where I felt my brain was no longer firing on all cylinders, and this resulted in many misfires. It is hard to explain the impact this had on me, especially because I had prided myself on perfection yet could no longer solve basic problems. I felt like I had lost a part of myself. I questioned the value I could have in the workplace if this was my new normal.

God gave me amazing abilities that I was able to use for decades, but I knew I would have to learn how to function in this world in a different way. I had no idea if I would regain my abilities or if my life was forever changed. It occurred to me how much I took these talents for granted and how much, in the past, I had not used them in a way that showed gratitude to the one who gave me my abilities. A seed was planted during my cancer journey that I should find another way to use my talents to help others. This yearning to do more with what I was given is the reason I left my job and focused on writing this book.

Being humble meant not only accepting my new normal with humor and grace but also being grateful and thankful for all God has given me. Embrace a key lesson cancer can bring, which is to understand what is truly valuable while modeling humility and using your talents to help others.

See Applying Insights in the Reflection & Action section to reflect more deeply on the insight that humility changes how we view life.

#10: Love
Seeing goodness in others
is transformative

More often than not, when we look at those around us, we look through a biased lens. We view and judge people and situations based on various filters, such as our experiences, attitudes, values, and beliefs. However, God sees each of us through his eyes of unconditional love. It doesn't matter what we have done, how we make a living, how much money we make, how educated we are, or what we look like. He loves each of us.

Have you ever had someone in your life who truly accepts you for you? This type of relationship provides unconditional support. You feel comfortable sharing your needs, wants, and desires with the individual. Despite what you have done, you know that person will always be there for you. Some of you have never had this type of relationship and may not be able to imagine how it feels to be in one. The closer you get to God, the more you will feel this type of support.

During my cancer journey, I was given another gift. God showed me how to see the goodness in people. He showed me how not to judge and to see beyond the harsh words or someone's actions to a deeper level of empathy than I had ever previously known. I often refer to this period of my cancer journey as the rose-colored-glasses phase.

For a funny take on this term, see the movie *Shallow Hal*. It is about someone who is judgmental and shallow but ends up falling in love with someone who is significantly overweight. After he experiences a transformation, he gains a new perspective and begins to see the inner beauty of the person rather than the outward appearance.

This is how I felt when I went back to work after I completed chemo and radiation therapies. I looked at people differently. All I could see was sheer goodness. This goodness radiated from each person, and I truly felt it. Whatever the individual did or said that may be perceived as negative didn't matter, as all I saw was a child of God.

At times, I couldn't remember people's names or recall having met someone. I learned to accept these mental blocks. I let go of any guilt and embarrassment as a result of this setback because I had no control over it. One senior leader was shocked that I could not recall meeting her multiple times. I got the sense she felt disrespected because she was such an important person in the organization. I actually felt sorry for her because her ego or self-esteem was so hurt by my lapse of memory, which showed a deeper issue that she must have been struggling with. Despite my poor memory, I had an increased ability to feel the pain of those I was communicating with.

My coworkers did not know the struggles I had with my mind. It made me realize how vital it was to remember, when interacting with others, that I may not know what the other person is going through, even if I felt their pain. If an individual spoke sharply or didn't follow through, I responded with grace.

I began to focus more on the individual rather than on the work in my interactions. When I heard people making negative comments about someone else, I tried to give them a different view to show the importance of empathy, humility, and support. Proverbs 16:24 (NLT) reminds us that "Kind words are like honey— / sweet to the soul and healthy for the body." I could feel, in some ways, the person's pain inside, which gave me a new appreciation for how to respond. I had a deeper level of empathy for the individual despite the persona they might have been displaying outwardly.

I remember feeling like this was a unique gift. I could see only the absolute good in people as Jesus did. I felt God's nonjudgmental and unconditional love for each person. It was so powerful and deeply moving to see people as good at their cores. It is difficult to describe the love I felt for others. It was so different from any feeling I had ever felt in the past, and I knew the Holy Spirit was showing me how God feels about each one of us—an all-encompassing love that is transformative.

I cherished every moment I felt this way. Because it was so impactful and deeply meaningful, I wondered how long it would last. I was aware at the time that God was giving me a glimpse of a perspective that was not permanent. I don't know why I thought this, but I now believe the Holy Spirit helped me see this was a temporary gift. Because I knew it was temporary, I consciously tracked how long this gift stayed with me.

I experienced this gift in full for about six months, and I thank God to this day for giving me the chance to see people differently. As time went on, the world's negativity started filtering back into my thinking, and my perspective shifted a bit. I now must work harder to focus only on the good when faced with negative people and situations, but this experience always comes back to remind me how life is more joyous, meaningful, and transformative when I'm focusing on the goodness of others and what it means to truly love my neighbor. I am thankful I kept a portion of this gift that lets me feel positive and negative influences when I speak with people, which allows me to identify those who may need my help, a listening ear, or an extra boost of encouragement or support.

I pray that you "may have the power to understand how broad and long, how high and deep, is Christ's love" for you (Ephesians 3:18 GNT). Once you understand how much God loves you, you will be able to share that love more freely with others. Ask God to show you his love and to help you see the goodness in all people. Ask him to help you approach every situation with unconditional love. It may be easier to look past the flaws of your loved ones and celebrate their goodness, but it's much harder to do this with people who are not as close. However, doing so will transform your life.

See Applying Insights in the Reflection & Action section to reflect more deeply on the insight that seeing goodness in others is transformative.

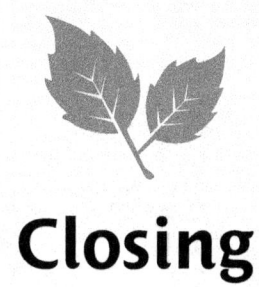

Closing

started this book by sharing that God gave me a gift. It is called cancer. God used my cancer journey to reshape my character and my perspective and to enrich my relationship with him. I believe God is using my experiences to give you hope and inspiration. My desire is that my words and life story have inspired you to remember that God loves you and wants to help you.

To realize the benefits I have shared, you must take action to change your point of view, including what you focus on and who and what you glorify. I have summarized key takeaways to help you transform your life through faith, hope, and love.

1. Foster and nurture a connection with God, giving him reverence and showing gratitude. Ask for God's help in every aspect of your life. Reflect on the blessings that are around you and thank him for them.

2. When you look at the world God has created, you can see that God loves diversity, yet each piece in the system has a role that contributes to the whole. Each of us has a broader purpose than just living for ourselves. Your cancer journey may be your opportunity to find out what that plan is. Life and our circumstances have a way of distracting us from what matters most. Mark 4:19 (GNT) reminds us, "The worries about this life, the love for riches, and all other kinds of desires crowd in and choke the message, and they don't bear fruit." As you face your health challenge, always remember that your life is a gift, and you can use your cancer journey to fulfill a broader purpose.

3. Review and reflect on the Testimonials and Insights and utilize Applying Insights resource as your guide. These are key tools to help with your transformation.

4. Refocus your thoughts on what really counts by fully embracing the fruit of the Spirit highlighted in Galatians 5:22–23 (GNT): "love, joy, peace, patience, kindness, goodness, faithfulness, humility, and self-control." Use the Behavior Positivity Tracker and Behavior Action Examples in the next section to bring attention to your behaviors.

5. Embrace nature to help you heal. God created the world in its natural form to be absolutely beautiful, and it is a present for us to enjoy and take care of. Nature has a way of rejuvenating the mind, body, and soul, aiding in recovery.

6. Review the Recommended Reading list toward the end of the book to discover new ways of approaching food and nutrition that could save your life by reversing your cancer or, at the very least, making you feel better. God gave us natural food that not only nourishes our bodies but also helps us heal if we are wise about what we eat.

7. Hydrate, hydrate, hydrate, and exercise. These need to be a key focus of your plan, not afterthoughts.

8. Write down key insights from your experiences as you implement changes. These lessons of life are powerful. They will help you to deepen your perception of your progress and remain focused on the blessings happening in your life. They will provide a platform for you to share these insights with someone else who may need your assistance.

Lastly, feel free to visit PenelopeCortez.com and share what God is doing in your life as a result of reading this book.

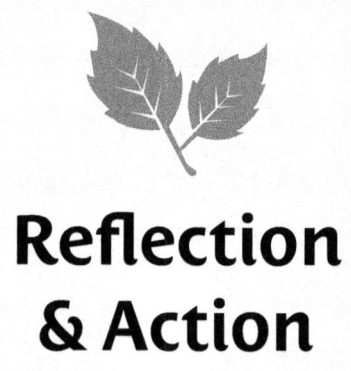

Reflection
& Action

Applying Insights

This section will help you reflect on and internalize the concepts discussed in Testimonials & Insights. I have provided Bible verses you may rely on as you deepen your understanding and begin to apply the ideas to your life.

Although I am not a Bible or spiritual expert, I found these verses meaningful. You may find other verses calling out to you as you explore a broader meaning for your life. This is how God works. He uses his Word in ways that relate to what you need at the right time, so each person may find some of the verses impactful based on what they are going through. I included a variety of verses in the hope that God will reach you based on what you need right now.

As you read through this section, consider copying some of the verses that most affect you to an Inspiration Log, which is available later in the section.

Testimonial Insight #1

Mindset:
Cancer doesn't define you

Trials

CONTEXT

Trials test our faith in what we believe and can help our characters grow. During any life challenge, you have a choice to humble yourself before God and ask for help. If you have faith, God will give you strength and endurance while changing your perspective along the way.

BIBLE REFERENCES

1 Corinthians 10:13 (GNT)

"Every test that you have experienced is the kind that normally comes to people. But God keeps his promise, and he will not allow you to be tested beyond your power to remain firm; at the time you are put to the test, he will give you the strength to endure it, and so provide you with a way out."

James 1:2–3 (GNT)

"My friends, consider yourselves fortunate when all kinds of trials come your way, for you know that when your faith succeeds in facing such trials, the result is the ability to endure."

Romans 12:12 (ESV)

"Rejoice in hope, be patient in tribulation, be constant in prayer."

REFLECTION

Think about where you are in your relationship with God. Being in a relationship with God is a choice. Are you angry with God for what is occurring in your life? Are you ignoring him because you don't believe in him or feel you do not deserve his help? Do you want his help to give you more strength and perseverance?

No matter where you are on this spectrum, take time to reflect on what it means to have a connection with God. Share your thoughts with God in prayer, including any concerns and feelings of uncertainty you may have with understanding what it means to have a relationship with him. Humble yourself by asking God to give you strength and endurance in your cancer battle, even though you may not fully know him yet. Ask God to use cancer as a way to grow your faith in him.

Mindset:
Cancer doesn't define you

Focus

CONTEXT

By focusing on God and his plan for your life, you will remove the distractions that are affecting your mental, emotional, physical, and spiritual health and begin to view cancer differently.

BIBLE REFERENCES

Colossians 3:2 (NIV)
"Set your minds on things above, not on earthly things."

Jeremiah 29:11 (GNT)
"I alone know the plans I have for you, plans to bring you prosperity and not disaster, plans to bring about the future you hope for."

Isaiah 41:10 (NLT)
"Don't be afraid, for I am with you. / Don't be discouraged, for I am your God. / I will strengthen you and help you. / I will hold you up with my victorious right hand."

REFLECTION

Today, make a commitment not to be a prisoner; don't allow cancer to take full control over your life. Don't let cancer rob you of the goodness that is already in your life. Remind yourself that you do not need to be afraid of cancer. Rather than dwell on your challenges, shift your focus. Celebrate what you have instead of thinking about what you don't have.

Start each day by reflecting on the goodness in your life, and do this before and after each treatment, as well. As you reflect, take a moment to glorify God and show him gratitude for these blessings. The more goodness you look for in your daily interactions, the more you will find.

Think about how your response to cancer, rather than cancer itself, can define you. As you reshape what you think about, you will have a deeper appreciation for and gratitude toward God and the people around you. You will become humble as you focus on what matters, and you will experience more peace and joy despite your current circumstances.

Testimonial Insight #1 (continued)

Mindset:
Cancer doesn't define you

God's Plan

CONTEXT

Although your cancer outcome is unclear, you must have faith that God is with you. Faith means trusting God's plan because he loves you unconditionally. Faith doesn't mean you will not have trials but that God can use these trials to show you his goodness and grace.

BIBLE REFERENCES

Proverbs 3:5–6 (NLT)
"Trust in the Lord with all your heart; / do not depend on your own understanding. / Seek his will in all you do, / and he will show you which path to take."

Romans 8:28 (GNT)
"We know that in all things God works for good with those who love him, those whom he has called according to his purpose."

Proverbs 16:9 (NIV)
"In their hearts humans plan their course, / but the Lord establishes their steps."

REFLECTION

Are you feeling that your life is out of control? Are you searching for a deeper understanding of your health challenges? In prayer, ask God to help you trust him and to help you see the good in your situation. Keep in mind that faith doesn't mean God will always answer your prayer requests during the time or in the way you expect. You must have faith that God is all-knowing and will only do what is best for you. Keep petitioning, but also be open to him providing a different response than what you asked for.

God has a purpose for your life that not only benefits you but also reinforces and glorifies him. It's an amazing feeling when you realize that you have a role in God's story. Ask God in prayer to show you what he wants you to learn and to help you align your actions and behaviors with his plan so that you may glorify him. Pray for God's help, strength, and support as you deepen your faith and trust in his plan for your life.

Testimonial Insight #2

Character:
Managing emotion grows character

Negative Emotions

CONTEXT

Negative emotions—such as anger, fear, and frustration—can lead to aggression, bitterness, depression, isolation, and despair if they are not managed. Negative feelings, if left unchecked, can impact recovery, whereas managing unpleasant emotions grows character and increases resiliency.

BIBLE REFERENCES

Ephesians 4:31–32 (GNT)
"Get rid of all bitterness, passion, and anger. No more shouting or insults, no more hateful feelings of any sort. Instead, be kind and tender-hearted to one another, and forgive one another, as God has forgiven you through Christ."

Philippians 4:8 (GNT)
"Fill your minds with those things that are good and that deserve praise: things that are true, noble, right, pure, lovely, and honorable."

Proverbs 19:11 (GNT)
"If you are sensible, you will control your temper. When someone wrongs you, it is a great virtue to ignore it."

REFLECTION

Think about a recent situation when you became impatient, angry, or sad. Reflect on why you felt that way or responded as you did. Consider any triggers that may have evoked the feeling or response, e.g., were you tired, did you feel ignored, or were you frustrated?

Ask God for help in making you aware of any triggers or root causes that could be contributing to your negative responses so you can recognize them when they happen in the future. When you are in a situation where unpleasant emotions are triggered, take a moment to pause and breathe. Think about these verses, and ask God to help you respond differently.

Keep a journal of the number of times you stopped yourself from reacting negatively. Reflect on how small changes in your responses affect you and those around you. Are you happier, more content, or less stressed? Do you have a more positive outlook on life?

Character:
Managing emotion grows character

Spiritual Characteristics

CONTEXT

Change is hard, and your will and determination will get you only so far. The Holy Spirit can help grow your character and provide you with the foundation to transform yourself into God's image during your cancer battle.

BIBLE REFERENCES

Ezekiel 36:26 (NIV)

"I will give you a new heart and put a new spirit in you; I will remove from you your heart of stone and give you a heart of flesh."

Galatians 5:22–23 (GNT)

"But the Spirit produces love, joy, peace, patience, kindness, goodness, faithfulness, humility, and self-control."

Romans 12:2 (NLT)

"Don't copy the behavior and customs of this world, but let God transform you into a new person by changing the way you think. Then you will learn to know God's will for you, which is good and pleasing and perfect."

REFLECTION

Review Galatians 5:22–23 and select at least two characteristics or behaviors you are struggling with. Make a list of actions you can take to demonstrate these traits. For example, how can you show love to a family member who is irritating you? How can you show kindness to a stranger? Practice implementing these behaviors and actions for at least two weeks.

While doing so, ask the Holy Spirit for help in transforming your character so your actions reflect his will for the changes you make. After two weeks, reflect on how you have changed and express gratitude to God for any positive effects.

In areas where you haven't changed, reflect on what that means. Is there a deeper reason that is driving you to behave in such a way? Have you been open with God about what that might mean? Continue praying about your growth and taking the necessary steps to transform your character to honor God. Although we can change when we have the desire and determination to, it is only through God's grace that we can fully transform into the person he wants us to be.

Look for the Behavior Positivity Tracker at the end of this section to help you keep track of the characteristics you want to change.

Testimonial Insight #3

Faith:
I am not alone

Your Protector

CONTEXT

No matter what you are facing, God is with you. He is your protector. No one is more powerful than God, and through him all is possible. Your faith in him will give you the strength and support to address your fears and challenges.

BIBLE REFERENCES

Deuteronomy 31:6 (NIV)
"Be strong and courageous. Do not be afraid or terrified because of them, for the Lord your God goes with you; he will never leave you nor forsake you."

Psalm 18:2 (GNT)
"The Lord is my protector; / he is my strong fortress. / My God is my protection, / and with him I am safe. / He protects me like a shield; / he defends me and keeps me safe."

Psalm 121:7 (NLT)
"The Lord keeps you from all harm / and watches over your life."

REFLECTION

Cancer and its associated treatments may make your body weak, but faith in God can make you strong despite your situation. When you become afraid or discouraged, think about the promises God made to you by reflecting on these verses. You are never alone when you are a child of God. As your father, God will protect and guide you.

Think about what it means to have a spiritual father who is there for you. Reflect on what it means to be protected and what you need from your defender. Humbly ask God in prayer to be your protector so you can be powerful and courageous. Thank God for the strength he will provide you, and faithfully believe he will do as he says. Remember, God is always holy and true to his Word.

Testimonial Insight #3 (continued)

Faith:
I am not alone

Burdens

CONTEXT

Worrying will not change the outcome. Scripture reinforces that God wants you to turn over your concerns to him. When you worry, it shows you are not trusting him because you do not have faith that he will take care of your needs.

BIBLE REFERENCES

Matthew 11:28–29 (NLT)
"Come to me, all of you who are weary and carry heavy burdens, and I will give you rest. Take my yoke upon you. Let me teach you, because I am humble and gentle at heart, and you will find rest for your souls."

1 Peter 5:7 (GNT)
"Leave all your worries with him, because he cares for you."

Psalm 55:22 (NLT)
"Give your burdens to the Lord, / and he will take care of you. / He will not permit the godly to slip and fall."

REFLECTION

It is difficult not to worry as you navigate your cancer battle, and it will take a focused effort and faith to release your concerns to God. Identify those areas you are most worried about. Then, re-read the verses provided. Reflect on the assurance that God is all-powerful and has way more resources and methods to solve problems than you do.

Share with God, in prayer, the difficulties you may have with letting go and allowing him to control the outcome. Ask God for help to open your heart and increase your faith so you can give your burdens to him.

If you release your worries to God—in your heart not just in your words—you will feel a weight lifted off your shoulders. When you feel your burdens being lifted, give praise and glory to him. Then watch the amazing blessings that will unfold.

Write down how it feels to have your burden lifted and what it means to you when it occurs so you do not forget the meaning of what transpired. You will begin to understand the importance of trusting God in all aspects of your life. Through this experience, you will know that God can and will take hold of your burdens so you do not have to carry them alone.

Testimonial Insight #3 (continued)

Faith:
I am not alone

Other Relationships

CONTEXT

Each of us has different talents, and we need each other to navigate life's challenges. God purposefully surrounds us with a unique community. Utilize your personal relationships to build a support network you can rely on and find comfort in.

BIBLE REFERENCES

Ecclesiastes 4:10 (BSB)

"For if one falls down, his companion can lift him up."

Galatians 6:2 (NIV)

"Carry each other's burdens, and in this way you will fulfill the law of Christ."

1 Thessalonians 5:11 (GNT)

"And so encourage one another and help one another, just as you are now doing."

1 Peter 4:10 (GNT)

"Each one, as a good manager of God's different gifts, must use for the good of others the special gift he has received from God."

REFLECTION

God intended for you to utilize those around you to help you. In fact, he commands us to help each other in times of need, as shown in the verses provided.

Reflect on any of your support needs that are not being met right now. Think about your broad network that can be used to provide you with more support. Do you have a friend or family member you trust with your innermost thoughts? Have you leaned on them to give you emotional support? Has someone already reached out with an offer to help? Instead of thinking you are burdening someone by asking for help, consider that you are giving them a gift by letting them serve and care for you.

In prayer, share your support needs with God, and humbly ask him to show you how the people in your life can help you meet those needs.

Testimonial Insight #4

Empathy:
Caring for others brings joy

Needs of Others

CONTEXT

Opportunities to assist others are presented every day. Remove the distractions and focus on what matters to truly see the needs around you. Helping others can have a positive impact on spiritual and emotional health and is a key part of loving thy neighbor.

BIBLE REFERENCES

Hebrews 13:16 (GNT)
"Do not forget to do good and to help one another, because these are the sacrifices that please God."

Romans 12:13 (NLT)
"When God's people are in need, be ready to help them. Always be eager to practice hospitality."

Acts 20:35 (GNT)
"I have shown you in all things that by working hard in this way we must help the weak, remembering the words that the Lord Jesus himself said, 'There is more happiness in giving than in receiving.'"

REFLECTION

Take a moment to think about the last time you looked at someone you didn't know with care and concern. How many times have you looked away or ignored someone who might need your help? Have you asked a family member or friend how he or she is doing and actually listened rather than just asking as part of a normal greeting?

Ask God to open your heart to the needs of those around you. Be more conscious and less distracted when interacting with others, and look for opportunities to help. Ask God to use you and your talents and resources in ways that align with his plan.

As you become more aware of the needs around you and take action to assist others, your perspective (what you think about, what you focus on, where you spend your time) will shift, and you will be blessed with more joy and happiness despite the challenges of cancer.

Testimonial Insight #4 (continued)

Empathy:
Caring for others brings joy

Kindness

CONTEXT

In Scripture, God reinforces the importance of kindness, and Jesus used kindness throughout his ministry. Research studies confirm that being kind can have significant benefits, including stress reduction and improvements in overall health and happiness.[21, 22]

BIBLE REFERENCES

Luke 6:27–28 (GNT)

"But I tell you who hear me: Love your enemies, do good to those who hate you, bless those who curse you, and pray for those who mistreat you."

Luke 6:31 (GNT)

"Do for others just what you want them to do for you."

Proverbs 11:17 (GNT)

"You do yourself a favor when you are kind. If you are cruel, you only hurt yourself."

Proverbs 21:21 (GNT)

"Be kind and honest and you will live a long life; others will respect you and treat you fairly."

REFLECTION

Reflect on what kindness means to you and how you demonstrate kindness in your daily interactions. Start with your own family. In the last week, identify examples of when you were kind and when you were unkind. Think about what led to each situation and what you would do the same or differently.

Humbly ask God in prayer for forgiveness for your unkind actions, and thank him for giving you the opportunity to display kindness. Tell those who you were not nice to that you are sorry and ask for their forgiveness. Think about easy changes you can make in your daily life to show more kindness to others.

Social media is a great test of Christian values. If you want to post unkind words publicly, ask yourself why you feel the need to do this. This could be a test of your faith. Do you trust God will right wrongs? The old adage that suggests you praise in public and correct in private is a good rule to live by. When you are faced with the opportunity to make an unkind comment, stop and ask God to give you wisdom and open your heart to act with kindness.

Testimonial Insight #4 (continued)

Empathy:
Caring for others brings joy

Taking Action

CONTEXT

It is easy to say you want to help others but much harder to actually act upon those desires, especially when you are not feeling well. Your illness should not be used as an excuse to not take action; instead, use it as a testimony to love your neighbor despite your setbacks. Through actions, you will discover true peace and joy.

BIBLE REFERENCES

James 1:22 (GNT)
"Do not deceive yourselves by just listening to his word; instead, put it into practice."

James 2:14 (NLT)
"What good is it, dear brothers and sisters, if you say you have faith but don't show it by your actions? Can that kind of faith save anyone?"

1 John 3:18 (GNT)
"My children, our love should not be just words and talk; it must be true love, which shows itself in action."

REFLECTION

Think about the broader needs in your community and the talents God gave you. How can you use your gifts and skills to meet the needs of others? Develop a list of actions you can take now and in the future that will help another person. The reality is that you may not be able to do what you envision right now, but you can take small steps. Don't create a barrier to helping because you don't think you can handle the full breadth of actions you have identified. Small steps in faith through actions are more important than a grandiose plan that is never implemented.

Once you have noted ways to help, pray about them. Ask God to help you focus on the highest priority actions, and be open to his response. He may give you tasks that aren't even on your list. Ask him to remove any barriers that prevent you from taking a step to help another. When you take the first step, glorify him for helping you act in ways that are aligned with his plan for you.

Testimonial Insight #5

Petition:
Prayer is powerful and comforting

Prayer

CONTEXT

Prayer is the mechanism to talk to God directly. It gives you a platform to honor and glorify him, understand his will for your life, increase your faith in him, ask for his guidance and support, share your struggles, and petition for what you need. Through prayer, you will be comforted and experience an increased sense of peace.

BIBLE REFERENCES

Colossians 4:2 (NLT)
"Devote yourselves to prayer with an alert mind and a thankful heart."

Philippians 4:6–7 (GNT)
"Don't worry about anything, but in all your prayers ask God for what you need, always asking him with a thankful heart. And God's peace, which is far beyond human understanding, will keep your hearts and minds safe in union in Christ Jesus."

Psalm 103:2–3 (GNT)
"Praise the Lord, my soul, / and do not forget how kind he is. / He forgives all my sins / and heals all my diseases."

1 Thessalonians 5:16–17 (NLT)
"Always be joyful. Never stop praying."

REFLECTION

How often do you pray? Do you only pray when you want something? When was the last time you thanked God for the blessings you have or expressed awe or admiration for what God has made and done for you? Take a moment to write down all your blessings. Honor God in prayer by thanking him for the goodness he has provided in your life.

Next, think about areas where you need forgiveness from the previous day or week and ask him for forgiveness. Now you are ready to share your concerns or requests, as you have humbled your heart.

Petition God for what you need and for his help in aligning your focus and actions with his plan. Have absolute faith that God is listening and he knows what you need before you even ask. Write down your petitions so you can keep track of your requests. Be open to how he answers your prayers, as it may not be how you expect. When God does answer, give him all the glory.

Testimonial Insight #5 (continued)

Petition:
Prayer is powerful and comforting

Faith

CONTEXT

Prayer without faith is worthless. When you have faith, the possibilities are endless. Be bold in your petitions while you pray because you know God is loving, merciful, and powerful. You must trust in God and believe he has your best interest at heart.

BIBLE REFERENCES

2 Corinthians 3:12 (GNT)
"Because we have this hope, we are very bold."

Hebrews 11:1 (NIV)
"Now faith is confidence in what we hope for and assurance about what we do not see."

Luke 1:37 (GNT)
"For there is nothing that God cannot do."

Mark 9:23–24 (GNT)
"'Everything is possible for the person who has faith.' The father at once cried out, 'I do have faith, but not enough. Help me have more!'"

REFLECTION

Recognize that prayer is not just about what you want but what God wants for you. His power and access to resources are unlimited, and he can solve problems in ways you have never even imagined. Just look at the book of Exodus and how God solved a problem the Israelites had as they escaped from bondage. No one could have predicted that Moses would part the Red Sea to allow the Israelites to get away from the Egyptians.

If you believe in God's power, there is no reason not to be bold in asking for what you need while recognizing the first priority needs to be God's will for your life. Aligning your requests with his plans will produce amazing results.

Think about where you are in your faith journey. In what ways are you showing a lack of faith in God's ability to help you? If you truly believe God can solve whatever issue you are dealing with, what would you say to him? How would it change your approach to life? Pray for more faith so you can make your requests with boldness. God doesn't expect us to be perfect, but he does want to hear from you so he can help you grow your faith in him.

Testimonial Insight #5 (continued)

Petition:
Prayer is powerful and comforting

Collective Prayer

CONTEXT

A key way to petition God for help is to ask others to pray with you. God wants his family members to support each other and pray for each other in collective prayer. Group prayer will bring another level of support that you need.

BIBLE REFERENCES

James 5:14 (GNT)

"Are any among you sick? They should send for the church elders, who will pray for them and rub olive oil on them in the name of the Lord."

James 5:16 (GNT)

"So then, confess your sins to one another and pray for one another, so that you will be healed. The prayer of a good person has a powerful effect."

Matthew 18:19–20 (GNT)

"And I tell you more: whenever two of you on earth agree about anything you pray for, it will be done for you by my Father in heaven. For where two or three come together in my name, I am there with them."

REFLECTION

Reflect on the verse that reminds us that when two or more people are gathered, God is listening. Have you asked others to pray for you? Why or why not? Reflect on the barriers stopping you from asking people to pray for you.

Group prayer can provide a deeper level of connection with God as others petition collectively on your behalf. Start with your family and friends, and ask them to pray for you. You can periodically send specific prayer requests based on the challenges or circumstances you are facing. This is a great way to allow others to help you while receiving the benefits of group prayer. You can formalize it by creating a small prayer team that meets periodically and prays together. With deep appreciation, thank those praying for you.

You can also ask your church or other ministries, such as K-LOVE, to pray for you. These ministries may also have support or prayer groups that you could join. Take some time to research the options available to you.

Testimonial Insight #6

Guidance:
God speaks to us in many ways

His Word (Scripture)

CONTEXT

The Bible contains information to guide your life. Reading the Bible will deepen your understanding of God, what he wants for you, and what he expects from you.

BIBLE REFERENCES

Hebrews 4:12 (GNT)
"The word of God is alive and active, sharper than any double-edged sword. It cuts all the way through, to where soul and spirit meet, to where joints and marrow come together. It judges the desires and thoughts of the heart."

Psalm 119:105 (GNT)
"Your word is a lamp to guide me / and a light for my path."

Romans 10:17 (ESV)
"So faith comes from hearing, and hearing through the word of Christ."

2 Timothy 3:16 (GNT)
"All Scripture is inspired by God and is useful for teaching the truth, rebuking error, correcting faults, and giving instruction for right living."

REFLECTION

Your first step in reading the Bible is to select a Bible translation that can help you understand God's message, as some Bible translations are harder to comprehend than others. I prefer the Good News Translation (GNT), as it uses common language. See the References section for a list of English Bible Translations. To help you select, choose one or two verses and compare and contrast the different translations. You can easily do this through online Bible study tools, such as Bible Hub.

Set aside five to ten minutes each morning to praise God and read the Bible. There are many free Bible applications, such as YouVersion and the BibleProject, that can guide you through a Bible reading plan. Another method is to think about a particular issue you are struggling with. Take time to research what the Bible says on the topic.

Be patient. The more you read, the more the Holy Spirit will unlock the meaning in the passages. In prayer, ask for help in interpreting verses you do not fully grasp. Use spiritual leaders to help you understand the messages. By reading the Bible, you will gain confidence in what God is saying, which will also help you avoid false teachings.

Testimonial Insight #6 (continued)

Guidance:
God speaks to us in many ways

Holy Spirit

CONTEXT

The Holy Spirit dwells in those who believe in Jesus, the Son of God. The Holy Spirit is a divine force that can guide you and influence your actions as you face difficult challenges in your life.

BIBLE REFERENCES

1 Corinthians 2:14 (GNT)

"Whoever does not have the Spirit cannot receive the gifts that come from God's Spirit. Such a person really does not understand them, and they seem to be nonsense, because their value can be judged only on a spiritual basis."

John 14:26 (GNT)

"The Helper, the Holy Spirit, whom the Father will send in my name, will teach you everything and make you remember all that I have told you."

Romans 8:27 (GNT)

"And God, who sees into our hearts, knows what the thought of the Spirit is; because the Spirit pleads with God on behalf of his people and in accordance with his will."

REFLECTION

The Holy Spirit enables you to have a personal relationship with God. Because the Holy Spirit is the Spirit of God living in you, you must believe in God and his Son to receive the Holy Spirit. As your guide and advocate, the Holy Spirit works in you to help you become the person God wants you to be if you allow him to do so.

Think about what it means to walk in partnership with God, Jesus, and the Holy Spirit. What areas of your life or your cancer battle could benefit from a guide or advocate working directly with you? If you are already a believer in God, were there times in your life when you felt compelled to take or not take action? If so, you may not have recognized that it was the Holy Spirit helping you. Affirm or reaffirm your belief in God and his son, Jesus. Ask the Holy Spirit in prayer what actions you need to take to receive the spiritual gifts that will transform you into the person God wants you to be.

Testimonial Insight #6 (continued)

Guidance:
God speaks to us in many ways

Other Ways

CONTEXT

God can speak to you in ways you may not initially recognize. As you grow in your spiritual maturity and deepen your faith, your heart and soul will be open to hear God more clearly in whatever communication venue he chooses.

BIBLE REFERENCES

2 Chronicles 5:14 (NLT)
"The priests could not continue their service because of the cloud, for the glorious presence of the Lord filled the Temple of God."

Isaiah 7:11 (GNT)
"Ask the Lord your God to give you a sign. It can be from deep in the world of the dead or from high up in heaven."

Job 33:14–17 (NLT)
"For God speaks again and again, / though people do not recognize it. / He speaks in dreams, in visions of the night, / when deep sleep falls on people / as they lie in their beds. / He whispers in their ears / and terrifies them with warnings. / He makes them turn from doing wrong; / he keeps them from pride."

REFLECTION

God may reach out to you to give you guidance, direction, encouragement, or correction. In this book, I highlighted various ways God spoke to me (people, books, Scripture, prayer, mini miracles, music, and nature). Every time I hear from God, it is a positive, life-changing experience. Be open to receiving and acting on God's wisdom. Always remember that God speaks through whatever or whomever he chooses but never in disagreement with the Bible.

Dreams, in particular, are hard to interpret. Leviticus 19:31 reminds us not to consult mediums, so if you have a dream, look to the Bible and Scripture experts to help you determine what the dream might mean.

In prayer today, ask God to give you the time, space, and awareness to pause, embrace, and appreciate the moments he shares his message with you. Ask God to open your heart to hear him and the Holy Spirit more directly so you can begin to see what he is trying to do in your life. God has a unique role for you, and discovering what that is will be life-changing. Write down any thoughts that come to mind as you reflect on this. Be patient and keep asking. As in any relationship, building trust takes time and nurturing.

Testimonial Insight #7

Support:
Resources are provided at the right time

Basic Needs

CONTEXT

For those who have faith, God will ensure your basic needs are met while you are battling cancer. This may include mental, physical, relational, financial, or spiritual needs.

BIBLE REFERENCES

2 Corinthians 9:8 (GNT)
"And God is able to give you more than you need, so that you will always have all you need for yourselves and more than enough for every good cause."

Matthew 6:33 (NLT)
"Seek the Kingdom of God above all else, and live righteously, and he will give you everything you need."

Philippians 4:19 (ESV)
"And my God will supply every need of yours according to his riches in glory in Christ Jesus."

Psalm 107:9 (ESV)
"For he satisfies the longing soul, and the hungry soul he fills with good things."

REFLECTION

First, express your gratitude to God in prayer for all that he has provided and what he will provide. Pray with confidence that he will deliver and meet your needs since Scripture reminds us of this truth.

Then, think about your basic needs that have not yet been met. Ask God for help in meeting these. We never know how God will meet our needs, but we must have faith that he will do so and at the appropriate time. When he meets your needs, give God praise with gratitude. If he doesn't, continue to petition for it or ask him to eliminate the need. Remember that God is not there to grant every want or desire you have. Because he knows what you really need and he has your best interests at heart, you must have faith that if your prayers are unanswered, there is a reason that you just do not understand.

Testimonial Insight #7 (continued)

Support:
Resources are provided at the right time

Timely Assistance

CONTEXT

God expects us to seek out trusted advisors to help us make decisions and utilize all his gifts and resources to navigate life's challenges at a time that is right and true.

BIBLE REFERENCES

Ecclesiastes 3:1 (GNT)
"Everything that happens in this world happens at the time God chooses."

Ecclesiastes 8:6 (NLT)
"For there is a time and a way for everything, even when a person is in trouble."

Proverbs 15:22 (NLT)
"Plans go wrong for lack of advice; / many advisers bring success."

Psalm 121:2 (GNT)
"My help will come from the Lord, / who made heaven and earth."

REFLECTION

Think about the decisions and risks you are managing as part of your cancer battle. What resources do you need to help you navigate this trial? Think broadly about resources. For example, resources may be financial, environmental, spiritual, human/people, or human-made. Can people, research, or organizations provide you with information to help you with decisions or minimizing risks? In what ways can you embrace nature or utilize natural resources? Are there financial programs that can assist you in your time of need? Think about all the people in your life who can help you build a plan to use all the resources God has given.

Ask God in prayer for help in identifying and providing the right resources to assist you at the times when you can best benefit from them. As resources are introduced to you, praise God for his goodness in giving you the resources at the right time.

Testimonial Insight #8

Forgiveness:
Grace gives us the power to forgive

Words

CONTEXT

There would be a lot less violence and hatred in the world if we were more thoughtful in our word choices. Harmful words can have lifelong consequences and can destroy relationships. If we control what we say, there will be less regret and a decreased need to ask for forgiveness.

BIBLE REFERENCES

Ephesians 4:29 (GNT)

"Do not use harmful words, but only helpful words, the kind that build up and provide what is needed, so that what you say will do good to those who hear you."

James 1:19 (GNT)

"Remember this, my dear friends! Everyone must be quick to listen, but slow to speak and slow to become angry."

Proverbs 15:1 (GNT)

"A gentle answer quiets anger, but a harsh one stirs it up."

Proverbs 21:23 (GNT)

"If you want to stay out of trouble, be careful what you say."

REFLECTION

Reflect on your recent conversations, and identify those individuals who may have made a hurtful comment to you. Ask God not to allow someone's misguided comments to have a negative impact on you and to help you respond with kindness, empathy, and compassion. Pray for the individual and ask God to address the issue that is causing that behavior.

When you catch yourself saying harmful words to others, pause and reflect on how you could express your views differently. Think about the verses provided and select different words that show kindness. In future interactions, strive to listen more and talk less as you connect with those you love. You will become wiser and more supportive of others in the process as you focus outwardly on the relationships rather than inwardly on what you want.

Ask God in prayer for help in making you more aware of how your words are affecting others. When you make a hurtful comment, be remorseful and humbly ask for forgiveness.

Testimonial Insight #8 (continued)

Forgiveness:
Grace gives us the power to forgive

Forgive

CONTEXT

Forgiveness doesn't mean you condone a behavior. Instead, you release any resentment and the ability to punish, hold judgment, or take vengeance, regardless of whether the individual actually deserves your forgiveness. It is through grace that you will be able to forgive so that you, too, can be forgiven.

BIBLE REFERENCES

Colossians 3:13 (NLT)
"Make allowance for each other's faults, and forgive anyone who offends you. Remember, the Lord forgave you, so you must forgive others."

Ephesians 4:32 (GNT)
"Instead, be kind and tender-hearted to one another, and forgive one another, as God has forgiven you through Christ."

Mark 11:25 (GNT)
"And when you stand and pray, forgive anything you may have against anyone, so that your Father in heaven will forgive the wrongs you have done."

REFLECTION

Think about an example of when you have hurt someone else. Contact the individual, apologize, and ask for forgiveness. Humbly ask God in prayer to help you repair the relationship. Once you have put in the effort to mend the hurt, release the burden and forgive yourself for the role you played in hurting another. If the individual cannot forgive you, pray for the person and allow God to work in their heart to heal any wounds.

Think about another example when someone hurt you, and you have not yet forgiven them. If you continue to carry resentment or bitterness, you can impact your health and recovery. Reach out to the person and share why you were so hurt by what happened. If the individual is remorseful, forgive with a humble heart. If not, ask God in prayer to take away your hurt so you can forgive the person. Trust that God will rectify any harm that may have been done.

Testimonial Insight #9

Gratitude:
Humility changes how we view life

The Provider

CONTEXT

All people and provisions come from God. It is essential for us to be grateful for what we have been given. As mentioned in Job 1:21, what the Lord gives, he can take away.

BIBLE REFERENCES

Ephesians 5:20 (NLT)
"And give thanks for everything to God the Father in the name of our Lord Jesus Christ."

James 1:17 (GNT)
"Every good gift and every perfect present comes from heaven; it comes down from God, the Creator of the heavenly lights, who does not change or cause darkness by turning."

Romans 11:36 (NLT)
"For everything comes from him and exists by his power and is intended for his glory. All glory to him forever! Amen."

1 Thessalonians 5:18 (NIV)
"Give thanks in all circumstances; for this is God's will for you in Christ Jesus."

REFLECTION

List the provisions in your life you think were provided by God and those provided by you. Reflect on the truth that everything comes from God. Focus on the provisions that you provided, and think about how God may have enabled each item. For example, you might have listed a home as something you have provided. Reflect on how God gave you talents, employment opportunities, and financial resources which provided the means to purchase the home.

After you go through this exercise, reflect on what God has done in your life to enable what you have. When was the last time you thanked God for the provisions on your list? If you were God, how would you feel if your child never thanked you? I am using human reasoning here to illustrate the point. However, we know God is more merciful than any of us. Think about how fortunate you are that God's love is unconditional.

Before asking God for a new set of wants, honor and glorify him for what he has provided. With humility, ask for forgiveness for not acknowledging his gifts to you. Thank him for deepening your understanding so you can recognize that all people and provisions come from him. Tell him you are deeply grateful for what he has given you.

Gratitude:
Humility changes how we view life

Value God and Others

CONTEXT

Cancer reminds us we cannot navigate life's challenges alone. Through a humble heart, we must give reverence to God and learn to value others above ourselves. This doesn't mean you are weak, unworthy, or beneath others, for we are all equal in God's eyes.

BIBLE REFERENCES

James 4:6 (NIV)

"But he gives us more grace. That is why Scripture says: / 'God opposes the proud / but shows favor to the humble.'"

James 4:10 (NIV)

"Humble yourselves before the Lord, and he will lift you up."

Luke 14:11 (GNT)

"For those who make themselves great will be humbled, and those who humble themselves will be made great."

Philippians 2:3 (NIV)

"Do nothing out of selfish ambition or vain conceit. Rather, in humility value others above yourselves."

Psalm 25:9 (NIV)

"He guides the humble in what is right and teaches them his way."

REFLECTION

Many of us go through life relying on ourselves. Self-reliance can be good in that you typically demonstrate perseverance and can adapt to situations; however, self-reliance can bring pride and arrogance and prevent you from realizing the full blessings and support that God wants to give you.

Think about any areas of your life where you find yourself boasting. Why do you feel the need to boast, be liked, be the center of attention, or feel insecure? How do you think your behavior impacts others? What message are you sending to God about his value when you boast?

Think of someone in your life who is humble. What do they do, how do they act, and what effect does that have on others?

Ask God in prayer to show you how to develop humility in the areas that will transform your character. Ask God for help and support to make the changes that will have the most impact so your behavior better aligns with the expectations he has for you, and so you may view life from a different perspective while you are battling cancer.

Testimonial Insight #10

Love:
Seeing goodness in others is transformative

Judgment

CONTEXT

We are all flawed, and only God can determine what is truly in a person's heart. Unrighteous judgment can cause more anxiety, stress, and depression and impact overall physical and mental health.

BIBLE REFERENCES

John 7:24 (NIV)

"Stop judging by mere appearances, but instead judge correctly."

Matthew 7:1–2 (GNT)

"Do not judge others, so that God will not judge you, for God will judge you in the same way you judge others, and he will apply to you the same rules you apply to others."

Matthew 7:3–5 (GNT)

"Why, then, do you look at the speck in your brother's eye and pay no attention to the log in your own eye? How dare you say to your brother, 'Please, let me take that speck out of your eye,' when you have a log in your own eye? You hypocrite! First take the log out of your own eye, and then you will be able to see clearly to take the speck out of your brother's eye."

REFLECTION

In today's world, many people feel compelled to share their opinion, and often these opinions are critical and judgmental. Sharing and acting on these are harmful to oneself, to the other party, and to society.

Think about recent examples of when you judged someone. What may be causing you to speak negatively about another person? In what ways have others judged you? Were there times when you were judged unfairly? How did this make you feel?

As you face your health challenges, you may become critical of others as you battle stress and uncertainty. When you find yourself judging another person unjustly, stop and say a quick prayer. Share with God that you understand it is not your place to judge others based on your standards and expectations. Plead for God's wisdom to help you respond to others based on his will. Maybe his will is to show mercy.

Write down the times you caught yourself judging someone. Thank God for raising your awareness so you can begin changing the way you respond to others.

Testimonial Insights #10 (continued)

Love:
Seeing goodness in others is transformative

Love Thy Neighbor

CONTEXT

Loving your neighbor can present rich opportunities for joy, peace, kindness, patience, and gratitude.

BIBLE REFERENCES

John 15:12 (NLT)

"This is my commandment: Love each other in the same way I have loved you."

Leviticus 19:18 (GNT)

"Do not take revenge on others or continue to hate them, but love your neighbors as you love yourself. I am the Lord."

1 Peter 4:8 (NLT)

"Most important of all, continue to show deep love for each other, for love covers a multitude of sins."

Romans 13:9 (GNT)

"The commandments, 'Do not commit adultery; do not commit murder; do not steal; do not desire what belongs to someone else'—all these, and any others besides, are summed up in the one command, 'Love your neighbor as you love yourself.'"

REFLECTION

Loving thy neighbor is an opportunity for you to adjust your focus from you and your situation to the needs of others. Loving your neighbor sounds easy, but in reality, it is difficult without God's help.

Reflect on these questions. Do you covet what someone else has? Are your biases about other people stopping you from seeing the goodness in them? Do you avoid someone who annoys you? Are you looking out for the welfare of others you may not know personally? Are you holding a grudge against someone? What barriers get in the way of loving your neighbor?

Despite your own challenges, you can take steps today to care for those around you. Ask God to open your heart to understand how you, with your unique talents and resources, can help others so you can honor his will. Take action and be a witness of how your life transforms as a result of loving your neighbor.

Behavior Positivity Tracker

In any life challenge, you may have negative behaviors as you become frustrated by your situation and the lack of control you have to change the outcome. The Positivity Tracker can help you adjust your actions through the identification and realization of how your behaviors are impacting you and those around you.

The characteristics highlighted in Galatians 5:22–23 are called the fruit of the Spirit. By demonstrating these traits with God's help, you will be a positive light to others you interact with, and you will change the way you look at life, your cancer battle, your relationships, and the world. You can use the tracker as a tally sheet to provide you with valuable information about reshaping your perspective, responses, actions, emotions, and feelings. However, it is only through God's help that you can truly transform. He knows what you need and can change your mind and heart to enable the transformation. Through Him, all is possible.

Positivity Tracker Instructions

This exercise involves tracking and reflecting on your characteristics, behaviors, emotions, and actions. For simplicity, I will refer to these collectively as *behaviors*.

+ Each column in the table can either reflect a specific day or week. Insert the date or week reference in the gray box at the top of each column.

+ When you demonstrate the behavior, place a tally mark in the appropriate box. For example, during your first week, if you felt joy, mark 1 in Column 1, Row B. Continue tracking the behaviors based on the time period you have designated.

+ At the end of the designated time period, write a total for each behavior in the respective box in Column 8.

+ Reflect on what the data is telling you. How did you impact others when you demonstrated each behavior? How did it affect you? What were your strengths? Where do you need more development?

+ Ask God for help in finding ways to utilize your strengths and to give you the wisdom to change those areas you identified as needing improvement.

+ As you make changes, reflect on how utilizing your strengths and adjusting to address behavioral gaps are altering your perspective. How is embracing the fruit of the Spirit transforming you? How has the Holy Spirit showed up to help you transform?

Refer to the Behavior Action Examples for a list of actions you can take to model the fruit of the Spirit.

Behavior Positivity Tracker

Fruit of the Spirit Galatians 5:22–23		Day or Week							Total
		1	2	3	4	5	6	7	Col. 8
Love	Row A								
Joy	Row B								
Peace	Row C								
Patience	Row D								
Kindness	Row E								
Goodness	Row F								
Faithfulness	Row G								
Humility	Row H								
Self-Control	Row I								

Behavior Action Examples

The Fruit of the Spirit Galatians 5:22–23	
Behavior	**Ways to Display**
Love	<ul><li>Send someone a personal note and express genuine concern or thanks.</li><li>Spend quality time with a family member or friend.</li></ul>
Joy	<ul><li>Laugh like no one is watching.</li><li>Cherish your time doing what you love.</li></ul>
Peace	<ul><li>Meditate on God's Word.</li><li>Spend time in nature and feel serenity.</li></ul>
Patience	<ul><li>Listen with the intent to understand.</li><li>Appreciate the value of the journey.</li></ul>
Kindness	<ul><li>Randomly help a stranger.</li><li>Volunteer your time or resources.</li></ul>
Goodness	<ul><li>Recognize a positive trait in another.</li><li>Do the right thing when no one is looking.</li></ul>
Faithfulness	<ul><li>Study the Word of God.</li><li>Glorify God for what he has done and will do for you.</li></ul>
Humility	<ul><li>Put someone else's needs before your own.</li><li>Thank God for the resources you have.</li></ul>
Self-Control	<ul><li>Do not react negatively to others. Hold your tongue.</li><li>Choose to eat foods to promote health.</li></ul>

Inspiration Log

Create a list of the top ten verses you can use to center your mind, body, and soul on God's Word. These verses are intended to bring you inspiration and hope and are a reminder that God is with you. You can choose from the verses provided or identify others you have found that encourage you and help you feel optimistic. Recite and reflect on these verses during your daily prayer time and before your treatments.

	Verse #	Verse
1		
2		
3		
4		
5		
6		
7		
8		
9		
10		

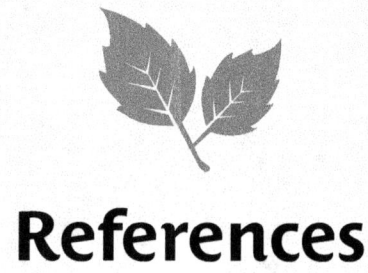

References

Recommended Reading

The following books helped me in my cancer journey. Updated versions of these materials may be available.

- Contreras, Francisco, and Daniel Kennedy. *Beating Cancer: 20 Natural, Spiritual, & Medical Remedies.* Lake Mary: Siloam, 2010.

- Fuhrman, Joel. *Super Immunity, The Essential Nutrition Guide for Boosting Your Body's Defenses to Live Longer, Stronger and Disease Free.* New York: HarperCollins, 2011.

- Keane, Maureen, and Daniella Chace. *What to Eat if You Have Cancer: Healing Foods That Boost Your Immune System.* New York: McGraw-Hill Books, 2007.

- Kushi, Michio, and Alex Jack. *The Cancer Prevention Diet: The Macrobiotic Approach to Preventing and Relieving Cancer.* New York: St. Martin's Griffin, 2009.

- Love, Susan M., and Karen Lindsey. *Dr. Susan Love's Breast Book, 5th Edition.* Philadelphia: Da Capo Press, 2010.

- Mendes, Dena. *A Survivor's Guide to Kicking Cancer's Ass.* Carlsbad: Hay House, 2010.

- Quillin, Patrick, and Noreen Quillin. *Beating Cancer with Nutrition.* Carlsbad: Nutrition Times Press, Inc., 2001.

Bible Verse Bibliography

Old Testament Books:
2 Chronicles, Deuteronomy, Ecclesiastes, Exodus, Ezekiel, Genesis, Isaiah, Jeremiah, Job, Leviticus, Proverbs, Psalms

New Testament Books:
1 & 2 Corinthians, 1 John, 1 Peter, 1 Thessalonians, 2 Timothy, Acts, Colossians, Ephesians, Galatians, Hebrews, James, John, Luke, Mark, Matthew, Philippians, Revelation, Romans

References

English Bible Translations

The Bible is translated not only into different languages but also into different versions. I have included a sample list for reference.

Abbreviations	Translation Name
AMP	Amplified Bible
ASV	American Standard Version
BSB	Berean Standard Bible
CEV	Contemporary English Version
CSB	Christian Standard Bible
ESV	English Standard Version
GNT	Good News Translation
GW	God's Word Translation
HCSB	Holman Christian Standard Bible
KJV	King James Bible
NASB	New American Standard Bible
NET	New English Translation
NIV	New International Version
NKJV	New King James Version
NLT	New Living Translation
WBT	Webster's Bible Translation

Citations and Sources

1 "BRCA Gene Mutations: Cancer Risk and Genetic Testing," National Cancer Institute, reviewed November 19, 2020, https://www.cancer.gov/about-cancer/causes-prevention/genetics/brca-fact-sheet.

2 "Lymphedema," Susan G. Komen, updated April 12, 2024, https://www.komen.org/breast-cancer/survivorship/health-concerns/lymphedema/.

3 Chani Smith, "Cording: A Treatable Complication of Breast Cancer Surgery," *British Journal of General Practice* 69, no. 685 (August 2019): 395, https://doi.org/10.3399/bjgp19X704825.

4 "Key Statistics for Breast Cancer," American Cancer Society, updated January 17, 2024, https://www.cancer.org/cancer/types/breast-cancer/about/how-common-is-breast-cancer.html.

5 Rick Warren, "Living an Anointed Life – Part 3,"PastorRick.com, February 2, 2023.

6 "Other Breast Cancer Genes," National Breast Cancer Foundation, updated January 17, 2024, https://www.nationalbreastcancer.org/other-breast-cancer-genes.

7 "Bisphenol A (BPA)," National Institute of Environmental Health Sciences, accessed May 31, 2014, https://www.niehs.nih.gov/health/topics/agents/sya-bpa.

8 "Canned Food Market Basket Survey," Can Manufacturers Institute, accessed May 31, 2024, https://www.cancentral.com/wp-content/uploads/2023/01/CMI-Washington-State-Canned-Food-Market-Basket-Report-Raw-Data.pdf.

9 April Rubin, "World Health Organization Warns Against Using Artificial Sweeteners," *New York Times*, posted May 25, 2023, https://www.nytimes.com/2023/05/15/well/eat/sweeteners-weight-loss-who.html.

10 Kirtida R. Tandel, "Sugar substitutes: Health controversy over perceived benefits," *Journal of Pharmacology and Pharmacotherapeutics* 2, no. 4 (Oct-Dec. 2011): 236-243, https://www.ncbi. nlm.nih.gov/pmc/articles/PMC3198517/.

11 Jenna Fletcher, "What might help protect the liver during chemotherapy?" Medical News Today, posted May 19, 2023, https://www.medicalnewstoday.com/articles/how-to-protect-liver-during-chemotherapy#signs-of-damage.

12 Dominique Delmas, Jianbo Xiao, Anne Vejux, and Virginie Aires, "Silymarin and Cancer: A Dual Strategy in Both in Chemoprevention and Chemosensitivity," *Molecules* 25, no. 9, 2009 (May 2020): 1-23, https://www.ncbi.nlm.nih.gov/pmc/articles/PMC7248929/.

13 Veronica Wendy Setiawan, et al., "Allium vegetables and stomach cancer risk in China," *Asian Pacific Journal of Cancer Prevention* 6, no. 3 (Jul-Sep 2005): 387-95, https://pubmed.ncbi.nlm.nih.gov/16236005/.

14 "Physical Activity and the Person with Cancer," American Cancer Society, revised March 16, 2022, https://www.cancer.org/treatment/survivorship-during-and-after-treatment/be-healthy-after-treatment/physical-activity-and-the-cancer-patient.html.

15 Mathew P. White, Ian Alcock, James Grellier, et al., "Spending at least 120 minutes a week in nature is associated with good health and wellbeing," *Scientific Reports* 9 (2019), https://doi.org/10.1038/s41598-019-44097-3.

16 "Kübler-Ross Change Curve," Elisabeth Kübler-Ross Foundation, accessed May 31, 2024, https://www.ekrfoundation.org/5-stages-of-grief/change-curve/.

17 Mary Stevenson, "Footprints in the sand," Footprints In the Sand, written 1939, accessed May 31, 2024, https://footprintssandpoem.com/mary-stevenson-version-of-footprints-in-the-sand/.

18 K-LOVE, http://klove.com/.

References

19 Dana Christensen, Stephen Fierbaugh, Jean Fischer, et al., *365 Encouraging Verses of the Bible for Women* (Uhrichsville, Ohio: Barbour Publishing, Inc, 2014).

20 "Chemo Brain," National Cancer Institute, accessed May 31, 2024, https://www.cancer.gov/publications/dictionaries/cancer-terms/def/chemo-brain.

21 Steve Siegle, "The art of kindness," Mayo Clinic Health System, posted August 17, 2023, https://www.mayoclinichealthsystem.org/hometown-health/speaking-of-health/the-art-of-kindness.

22 Lee Rowland and Oliver Scott Curry, "A range of kindness activities boost happiness," *Journal of Social Psychology* 159, no. 3 (2019): 340-343, https://doi.org/10.1080/00224545.2018.1469461.

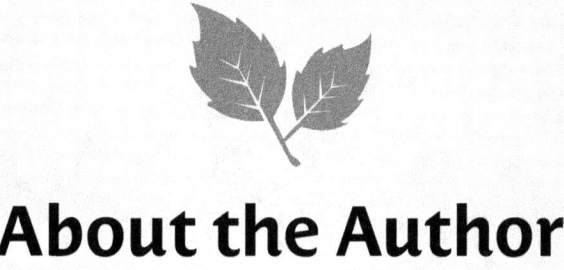

About the Author

Penelope Cortez is a seasoned business professional with a master's degree in business and more than three decades of corporate experience. Beyond her successful career, Penelope—known affectionately as Penny—is a writer, philanthropist, and the visionary founder and CEO of Levers4Change. Penny is also a devoted wife and mother of two daughters.

Her life took a profound turn when she was diagnosed with cancer, a journey which reshaped her perspective and deepened her faith in God. Through this challenging chapter, she gained invaluable insights that led her to embrace a divine calling to share her story. Romans 12:13 (NLT) reminds us, "When God's people are in need, be ready to help them." Inspired by this verse, Penny wrote this book as a beacon of hope, providing support and inspiration to those in need.

Through her writing and philanthropic efforts, Penny continues to empower others to navigate life's challenges with hope, resilience, and unwavering faith.